Coping and Prevention

A volume in
Stress and Quality of Working Life
Ana Maria Rossi, Pamela L. Perrewé, and James A. Meurs, *Series Editors*

Coping and Prevention

edited by

Ana Maria Rossi
International Stress Management Association

Pamela L. Perrewé
The Florida State University

James A. Meurs
University of Mississippi

IAP

INFORMATION AGE PUBLISHING, INC.
Charlotte, NC • www.infoagepub.com

Library of Congress Cataloging-in-Publication Data

Coping and prevention / edited by Ana Maria Rossi, Pamela L. Perrewi, James A. Meurs.
p. cm. – (Stress and quality of working life)
Includes bibliographical references.
ISBN 978-1-61735-701-5 (pbk.) – ISBN 978-1-61735-702-2 (hbk.) – ISBN 978-1-61735-703-9 (ebook)
1. Job stress. 2. Work–Psychological aspects. 3. Industrial psychiatry.
4. Psychology, Industrial. I. Rossi, Ana Maria. II. Perrewe, Pamela L.
III. Meurs, James A.
HF5548.85.C658 2012
158.7'2–dc23

2011045542

Printed and bound by CPI Group (UK) Ltd, Croydon, CR0 4YY

CONTENTS

SECTION II

EXAMINING IMBALANCE AND MISMATCH MODELS OF STRESS

SECTION III

THE ROLE OF THE ORGANIZATION AND QUALITY OF WORK LIFE IN STRESS

SECTION IV

EXAMINING THE BIGGER PICTURE OF OCCUPATIONAL HEALTH AND WELL BEING

FOREWORD

Occupational stressors are an unavoidable part of working life. Experiencing stress has helped us to survive for thousands of years and keeps us vigilant under critical situations. Of course, too much experienced stress can lead to serious psychological and physical health problems. This book is devoted to examining important issues related to coping with and preventing elevated occupational stress. This book also examines individual differences and organizational cultures that might exacerbate or mitigate experienced stress.

In the third volume of *Stress and Quality of Working Life,* we are pleased to present our book of readings entitled, "Coping and Prevention." We divide our book into four major sections. The first section, *The Role of the Individual in Occupational Stress,* includes four chapters. In the first chapter, Valentina Bruk-Lee and Paul Spector propose a model of how conflict at work is connected with strain. They pay particular attention to how personality and conflict management styles affect their perspective of workplace conflict. In the second chapter, Jason Stoner and Pamela Perrewé explain the role of identity in the workplace stress process. Their chapter details how individuals' identities influence perceptions of occupational stressors and how a person's identity hierarchies affect the use of social support. In the third chapter, Edilaine Silva Gherardi-Donato and colleagues examine the impact of individuals' alcohol use on work, general health, and well-being. In the fourth chapter, Jessica Streit, Steven Sauter, and Dennis Hanseman examine age-related trends in worker health and well being. They focus on the individual difference variable, age, and examine the evidence on risks of job stress and well being among older workers.

Coping and Prevention, pages ix–x

The second section, *Examining Imbalance and Mismatch Models of Stress,* includes two chapters. In Chapter 5, Johannes Siegrist identifies the importance of social reward in the stressful psychosocial environment of work. The chapter also reviews the empirical evidence linking an imbalance of effort and rewards at work with poor health and a heightened risk of stress-related physical and mental disorders, and discusses the managerial implications of this body of research. In Chapter 6, Chad Peddi and his colleagues consider the influence of an individual's regulatory focus on health. Their study demonstrates that having a mismatch between a person's chronic regulatory focus and state regulatory focus has negative health implications.

In the third section, *The Role of the Organization and Quality of Work Life in Stress,* we have five chapters examining different aspects of this important phenomenon. In Chapter 7, Kristi Zimmerman and her colleagues provide evidence for the importance of an organization's culture of social support. Specifically, they examine the influence of a family-supportive culture on the conflict between work and family and on the emotional exhaustion of teachers. The eighth chapter, by Tatiana Serverino de Vasconcelos, examines organizational work-life programs. Within the public security context, Vasconcelos examines stress management and occupational quality of life programs. In Chapter 9, Avelino Luiz Rodrigues and colleagues examine quality of life and burnout among an important segment of the population: physicians. Ieda Rhoden, in Chapter 10, examines ways to cope with hypermodern life by utilizing different facets of constructive spare time. Finally, this section includes Chapter 11 by Elizabeth P. Mendes Riberio and Sérgio Rocha, who also examine quality of life issues. Specifically, they examine women in modern times and the relation with quality of life.

Our final section four, *Examining the Bigger Picture of Occupational Health and Well Being,* includes three closing and overview chapters. In Chapter 12, Thomas Zeni, Mike Buckley, Anthony Klotz, and Milorad Novicevic identify threats to validity as they pertain to the study of leadership by highlighting the shortcomings of physiological stress research. Chapter 13, by Artur Zular, examines a psychosomatic view of people management. In our final chapter, Chapter 14, Joseph Hurrell and Steven Sauter present a comprehensive framework of job stress and health developed by researchers at the National Institute for Occupational Safety and Health. The chapter reviews the various factors that play a role in workplace stress and health.

We hope you enjoy the third volume of *Stress and Quality of Working Life: Coping and Prevention.* We believe we have an outstanding group of organizational scientists who, together, present an interesting, diverse, and cutting-edge perspective on stress, health, and well-being in occupational research.

—Ana Maria Rossi
Pamela L. Perrewé
James A. Meurs

PREFACE

The corporate environment—a place of continuous activity and demands—is considered one of the great villains of workers' health for triggering stress-related symptoms. The cost of stress at the workplace has been frequently calculated. Information published by The American Institute of Stress (AIS) shows that US$ 300 billion/year are spent on conditions related to excessive stress levels. The estimates in Brazil are that the loss corresponds to 3.5% of the GDP/year.

Occupational diseases are directly related to the activity performed by workers and to the working conditions in the company. In addition to affecting workers' health, they can also worsen existing symptoms. Among the occupational diseases are the technology-related diseases caused by work activities and the conditions related to excess effort.

If we consider all choices available, it is better to prevent than to treat. Prevention can be primary, when we prevent the stress-generating situation from occurring; secondary, when we provide alternatives to minimize the damage caused by the problem; and tertiary, which involves containing losses that have occurred to prevent them from becoming more serious.

Facing this reality, the purpose of ISMA-BR is to discuss studies and practices at the corporate level and warn about the importance of bringing together high productivity and an environment that promotes well-being and physical and mental health.

ISMA was established in Brazil in May 2000. Since then, it has been dedicated to the dissemination of scientific knowledge on the prevention and treatment of stress. It is considered a reference in professional training in Brazil and South America, conducting training courses, scientific research

Coping and Prevention, pages xi–xii

and making people aware of the importance of diagnosis, preventive actions, and proper treatment.

This book on stress coping and prevention is one additional initiative to mitigate the increasing levels of stress in the workplace. We believe that through the information and practice from lessons learned that are provided here by some recognized professionals in this field in the world we will be able to achieve the aspired balance. Reading this book is an important step towards making this goal come true. I wish you all a good reading and a less stressful life.

—Ana Maria Rossi, PhD
President of ISMA-BR

SECTION I

THE ROLE OF THE INDIVIDUAL IN OCCUPATIONAL STRESS

CHAPTER 1

INTERPERSONAL CONFLICT AND STRESS AT WORK

Implications for Employee Health and Well-Being

Valentina Bruk-Lee
Florida International University

Paul E. Spector
University of South Florida

In an ever-expanding and changing workplace, social interactions with others continue to play important functions, such as information sharing, goal attainment, and social networking. What happens, then, when conflict arises in the workplace where individuals or groups of individuals have disputes that can be disruptive and heated? What impact does it have on employee well-being and relevant organizational outcomes? What important factors moderate these relationships? This chapter will address these and related questions focusing primarily on the negative impact conflict might have on the well-being of employees who experience it.

Coping and Prevention, pages 3–22

Conflict at work is defined as a "dynamic process that occurs between parties as they experience negative emotional reactions to perceived disagreements and interference with the attainment of their goals" (adapted from Barki & Hartwick, 2001, p. 198). It can occur at the individual level between two people who might be from the same or different work groups. It can occur at the group level when group members band together against another group. It can also occur at the organizational level, for example, when organizations in the same industry sue one another over contract violations. While a comprehensive discussion of conflict would include antecedents, outcomes, and process variables at the various levels of analysis, the study of conflict related to well-being of employees has focused almost entirely on it as an interpersonal event.

Conflict taxonomies distinguish among conflict types (see Amason & Schweiger, 1994; Barki & Hartwick, 2004; Jehn, 1994; Pinkley, 1990). The most often-used distinction is between task and relationship conflict (Pinkley, 1990). Task conflict refers to conflict situations emerging from task-related issues, such as differing viewpoints regarding the goals of a work task. Relationship conflict refers to personality clashes and/or emotionally charged interactions with others due to issues of a personal nature. Recent research has identified two additional forms of conflict, although not much research has been done on either one. Jehn (1997) defined process conflict as instances of conflict regarding the procedures for completing a task, including how tasks should be performed, when, and by whom. This is distinguished from task conflict that is concerned with the goals of work tasks rather than the specific procedures used to achieve them. Lastly, non-task organizational conflict emerges from issues that are organizational in nature, but not specific to a work task, such as disagreements over workplace policies, benefits, and so on (Bruk-Lee, 2006).

The distinction between relationship and task conflict has shaped much of the business and communication research, which has focused on the differential impact of conflict types on relevant outcomes (see DeDreu & Weingart, 2003). Results supporting a positive relationship between moderate amounts of task conflict and organizational outcomes, such as decision quality, improved team performance, conception of new ideas, and effective use of resources, have served as the basis for the widely cited proposition that task conflict may be functional and desirable (Amason, 1996; Baron, 1991; Fiol, 1994; Jehn, 1994, 1995, 1997; Tjosvold, Dann, & Wong, 1992). Relationship conflict, on the contrary, has been posited as dysfunctional and detrimental to the work environment with research indicating a negative impact on performance, productivity, and satisfaction (De Dreu & Weingart, 2003; Jehn, 1994, 1995). However, recent academic debates and meta-analytic summaries of results across multiple studies have challenged these ideas by indicating that conflict, regardless of specific type, can have a negative effect on individuals in the workplace (De Dreu, 2008; De Dreu & Weingart, 2003).

Nevertheless, even if moderate amounts of task conflict can serve a beneficial role, findings indicate a positive association with relationship conflict (Simons & Peterson, 2000). This suggests that conflict types are not mutually exclusive and that, instead, they can evolve or escalate into various forms (Jehn, 1997; Amason & Schweigher, 1994). In other words, it might well be that task conflict, even if itself productive, can lead to harmful relationship conflict. Studies have found various moderator variables that likely increase the tendency for task conflict to lead to relationship conflict, including low levels of trust among people and high levels of ambiguity about people's expected roles (Simons & Peterson, 2000; Tidd, McIntyre & Friedman, 2004).

In addition to specific conflict types, some researchers have focused on the sources of conflict. Interpersonal sources are coworkers versus supervisors (Bruk-Lee & Spector, 2006; Frone, 2000), as well as clients, customers, and patients. Results from these studies support the notion that whom the conflict is with influences both the personal and organizational outcomes reported, such that conflicts with supervisors are more strongly related to outcomes of organizational relevance. De Dreu and Gelfand (2007) summarized three potential sources of conflict: conflict over limited resources and opposing interests, conflicts over one's values or threat to one's ego and self-view (i.e., relationship based), and conflicts over different interpretations of information.

A STRESS FRAMEWORK OF CONFLICT AT WORK

Conflict research can be categorized into multiple streams, one of which focuses on the emergence of conflict and its link to employee health and well-being. Taken from an occupational stress perspective, interpersonal conflict is a social stressor or a social condition that an individual will find stressful. These stressors have been linked to a variety of employee health and well-being outcomes, termed strains, that can be physical (e.g., cardiovascular disease or headaches), psychological (e.g., negative emotions such as anxiety or anger), and behavioral (e.g., alcohol consumption or smoking). Social stressors include many forms of adverse interactions among people in the workplace. The most mild form of social stressor is incivility in which an individual might find another to be rude and insensitive (Pearson, Andersson, & Porath, 2005). At the other extreme is physical violence in which an employee is assaulted by others—for example, nurses being assaulted by patients (Spector, Coulter, Stockwell, & Matz, 2007). Other forms of social stressors involve mistreatment of employees by coworkers and supervisors—for example, workplace bullying (Rayner & Keashly, 2005).

What distinguishes conflict from these other forms of social stressors is that conflict implies a two-way exchange among two or more parties rather than a more passive target being the recipient of hurtful treatment by one or more actors. There is, however, considerable overlap between conflict and other social stressors as incivility, verbal mistreatment, and even physical aggression can be involved during conflict. Furthermore, conflict can have very much the same relationship with employee well-being as other social stressors (Hershcovis, in press).

Early conceptualizations of conflict included structural models that emphasized the contextual factors surrounding conflict, such as the interdependence among parties. More recent process models, however, conceptualize conflict as a dynamic sequence of events and take into account not only the objective or structural conditions for conflict, but also the role of perceptions, emotion, and behavior. Spector and Bruk-Lee (2008) presented an emotion-centered model of conflict at work grounded in the stress literature and focused on the dynamic process by which conflict affects employee health and well-being (see Figure 1.1). Similar to other stress frameworks, the proposed model assumes a causal flow from perceived conflicts to resulting strains. Nonetheless, it recognizes that feedback loops may exists at various points of the process and that conflict is a dynamic and complex

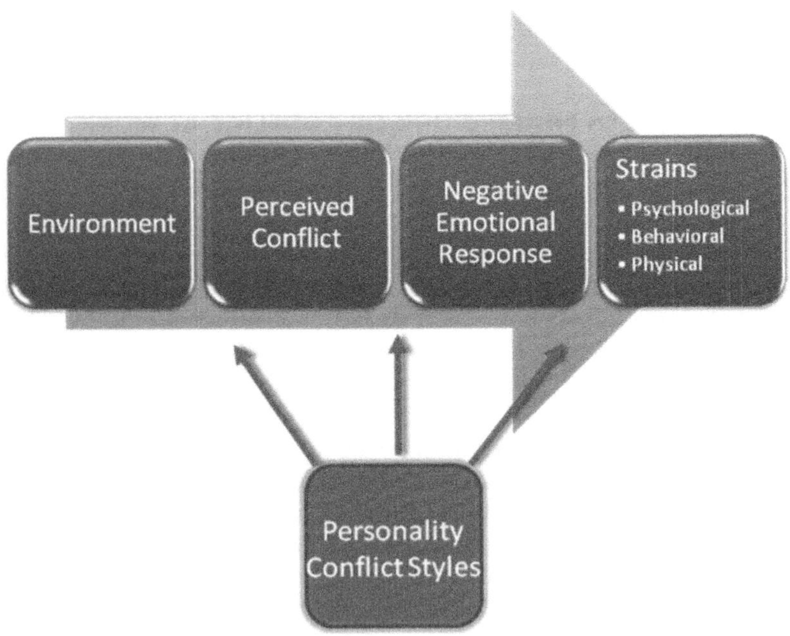

Figure 1.1 Stress based framework of conflict at work.

event. Perception plays an important role in the model, which depicts an interaction between the objective environment and personal characteristics in determining whether a specific incident is considered to be threatening and hence, a stressor (Lazarus, 1999).

The environmental conditions that may lead to perceived conflict are many. One such environmental factor is the current global economic crisis, which has resulted in company closures, layoffs, financial cutbacks, mergers, outsourcing, and an increasingly competitive job market for the growing percentage of the unemployed. Together, these conditions contribute to a tense social work environment where employees are expected to do more with fewer resources while dealing with a heightened sense of job insecurity. Rapid globalization has also increased the use of technologies that have changed the traditional channels and norms of communication and the social infrastructure of workgroups, as well as introduced diversity to organizations. These and other environmental conditions can present an opportunity for conflict among individuals within and outside an organization.

Interpersonal conflict at work may pose a threat to one's general desire for harmonious relationships, established routines, or preferred processes among other factors. Conflict can also interfere with one's attempts at goal achievement, thus reducing one's sense of control. Hence, when encountered, conflict incidents are likely to be perceived as stressors.

The model proposes that the immediate response to interpersonal conflict is negative emotion, perhaps most often anger, although anxiety, depression, and other emotions can also occur. Negative emotions can be part of an adaptive response and precede various forms of strains, which can be behavioral (calling in sick to avoid the person with whom one is having a conflict), physical (getting a tension headache), and psychological (losing commitment to the employer).

Conflict at work has been regarded as a leading source of occupational stress across nations. For example, when asked to describe the most stressful recent event at work, conflict is near the top of the list in China (Liu, Spector, & Shi, 2007), India (Narayanan, Menon, & Spector, 1999a), and the U.S. (Liu et al., 2007; Narayanan, Menon, & Spector, 1999b). The potential impact of this social stressor on well-being has also received attention by researchers in Greece (Lazuras, Rodafinos, Matsiggos, & Stamatoulakis, 2008), Japan (Inoue & Kawakami, 2010), the Netherlands (Giebels & Janssen, 2005; De Dreu, van Dierendonck, & Dijkstra, 2004), Spain (Guerra, Martinez, Munduate, & Medina, 2005), Finland (Appelberg, Romanov, Honkasalo, & Koskenvuo, 1991), and the United States (Bruk-Lee, Nixon, & Spector, submitted; Spector & Bruk-Lee, 2008; Spector & Jex, 1998), among others.

Much of the research on conflict as a social stressor has focused on relationship-based conflict as a function of the measures used in assessing its occurrence. Nonetheless, the few studies differentiating between conflict types suggest that all forms of conflict have significant relationships with well-being (Bruk-Lee et al., submitted; Bruk-Lee & Spector, 2006).

The remainder of this chapter will present a summary of research findings that link conflict to the three main strain types: psychological, physical, and behavioral. We will also discuss conditions that may affect the conflict–strain relationship with a special focus on the role of personality variables and individual conflict management styles. Last, practical implications are presented.

Psychological Well-Being and Conflict at Work

As noted in the conflict–stress model, the immediate strain response to conflict is negative emotion. This, perhaps, is not surprising considering the key role negative emotions plays in the conflict–strain process. Among the specific emotional strains studied are anger, anxiety, and depression, as well as more global measures of general negative mood and emotion. In fact, conflict incidents at work were among the strongest influences on psychological distress and daily mood (Bolger, DeLongis, Kessler, & Schilling, 1989).

Symptoms of depression have been widely reported in social stressor studies using both cross-sectional and longitudinal research designs (Dormann & Zapf, 1999, 2002). Both individual studies and meta-analyses that summarize results across multiple studies report that individuals who experience conflict will be more depressed than individuals who do not (Bruk-Lee, Nixon, Spector, 2010; Heinisch & Jex, 1997; Spector & Jex, 1998). These results extend to working samples outside of the United States, hence highlighting the importance and prevalence of conflict as a stressor cross-culturally. For example, relationship and task conflict have been shown to be associated with poor emotional well-being of workers in both private and public organizations in Spain (Guerra et al., 2005). Similarly, a study of over 20,000 Japanese employees in various manufacturing plants found relationships between intergroup conflict and depression for men (Inoue & Kawakami, 2010).

Similarly, anger (Spector & Jex, 1998) and anxiety (Bowling & Beehr, 2006) have been found to relate to conflict. Individuals who experience more conflict tend to be more anxious and angry than individuals who do not. That anger is related to conflict is not surprising since anger can be very much a part of conflict, and the expression of anger by two parties can contribute to conflict escalation. One might expect that anger would be inhibited when conflict involves a superior, and might instead be associated with anxiety over being punished or even fired as a result of such conflict.

Burnout is a state of emotional exhaustion and depersonalization that can be a strain response to an overly stressful job (Maslach, 1982). Research supports the influence of the social work environment on predicting feelings of burnout. In particular, employees in healthcare occupations or those dealing with the public appear to be at higher risk. Nurses, for example, report feelings of burnout in relation to increased interpersonal conflict with patients, peers, and supervisors (Abrahamson, Anderson, Anderson, Suitor, & Pillemer, 2010). Negative interpersonal interaction was also a predictor of burnout across samples of sports officials, public transportation drivers, and social workers (Giebels & Janssen, 2005; Rainey, 1995; van Dierendonck & Mevissen, 2002). The implications of these findings are important given the fact that burnout is associated with health symptoms and is a predictor of changes in cholesterol and triglycerides levels that can contribute to cardiovascular disease (Shirom, Westman, Shamai & Carel, 1997).

Among the most widely used indicators of psychological well being for employees is satisfaction with one's job or work group. Consistent findings indicate that employees who experience more task, relationship, or non-task organizational conflict at work also feel less satisfied (cf. Bruk-Lee, Nixon, & Spector, submitted; De Dreu & Weingart, 2003; Spector & Jex, 1998). These findings have been replicated with measures of both interpersonal and intragroup conflict and across a variety of occupations and nationalities.

Physical Health and Conflict at Work

Physical strains can be the byproduct of the occupational stress process. Short-term physical strains can be the physical component of negative emotion. Individuals experiencing anger or anxiety will undergo short-lived physiological reactions such as increased blood pressure or heart rate. Such responses can lead to more enduring physical changes that might result in physical symptoms such as headache or stomach distress. Long-term physical strains are stress-related illnesses including cardiovascular disease that can develop over many years of exposure to risk factors that include occupational stress.

The long-term implications of stress in general on cardiovascular health have received substantial attention. For example, longitudinal findings from the Work Site Blood Pressure study reported an increased risk of hypertension and increased ventricular mass for employees experiencing job stress (Schnall, Schwartz, Landsbergis, Warren, & Pickering, 1998). Nevertheless, the mechanisms underlying the association between stress and cardiovascular health are still unclear, and more research is needed to identify key psychosocial stressors and understand the ways in which they assert an influence on heart health (American Heart Association, 2010).

Laboratory and field studies show an association between social stressors (conflict at work) and heightened cardiovascular reactivity in both men and women. For example, Piferi and Lawler (2000) indicated that even low hostility women displayed heightened cardiovascular reactivity after an episode of interpersonal conflict. Similarly, women in a laboratory study reported a variety of negative emotions that were shown to impact elevations in heart rate and blood pressure after a conflict incident (Lavoie, Miller, Conway, & Fleet, 2001). In field studies, traffic enforcement officers displayed elevated blood pressure under conditions of negative interpersonal interactions, and the negative emotions experienced during such episodes were positively correlated with blood pressure (Brondolo, Karlin, Alexander, Bobrow, & Schwartz, 1999). In addition, problems with others at work were significantly related to higher blood pressure among a Dutch working sample (Van Dijkhuizen & Reiche, 1980).

Conflict's influence on physical health has also been studied using self-reports of physical symptoms, which are physical manifestations of psychological distress. Typically, studies use symptom checklists that ask employees to report the occurrence of headaches, stomach disorder, eye strain, and chest pain, among others. A consistent body of research, including two meta-analyses, supports the association between interpersonal conflict at work and reports of somatic symptoms (Nixon, Mazzola, Bauer, Krueger, & Spector, 2011; Spector & Jex, 1998). Employees experiencing more conflict in the workplace report more somatic symptoms. This relationship has also been found using qualitative data methods and in non-U.S samples (Hahn, 2000; Lazuras et al., 2009). Haug, Mykletun, and Dahl (2004) reported that patients with somatic symptoms have a high degree of disability compensation and tend to overuse the healthcare system. Similarly, in a study with over 15,000 employees, Appelberg, Romanov, Heikkila, Honkasalo, and Koskenvuo (1996) concluded that interpersonal conflict at work can be a significant determinant of work disability, particularly among women.

Behavioral Strains and Conflict at Work

People respond to stressors with a variety of behaviors, many of which have implications for both organizational and personal outcomes. Workplace accidents that can lead to injury, for example, can be the byproduct of behaviors that increase the likelihood of mishap. Accidents can occur because stressors lead to employees disregarding proper safety protocols, or because the distraction of stressors leads to errors that have tragic consequences. Dispositional and work environment factors have been studied in attempts to better understand employee behavior and effective ways to design safe work conditions (Smith, Karsh, Carayon, & Conway 2003; Shaw &

Sichel, 1971). Commonly studied stress variables, such as workload, managerial social support, and job dissatisfaction, have been shown to play a role in occupational injuries (Frone, 1998; Hemingway & Smith, 1999; Smith, Cohen, Cohen, & Cleveland, 1978). However, research on the impact of social stressors is scarce. Nonetheless, limited evidence suggests that interpersonal conflicts at work are positively related to workplace injuries. Frone (1998) tested a model of workplace accidents among employed adolescents in which interpersonal conflicts with supervisors and coworkers were both significantly correlated with a measure of job related injuries. Results from a study on employee drug usage also indicated conflicts at work were related to a significant probability of experiencing a job injury (Macdonald, 1995). Similarly, a review of the occupational stress and injury literature concluded that interpersonal disagreements with superiors and peers were statistically significant factors for accidents (Johnston, 1995). A more distal, but interesting, connection between conflict and accidents was proposed by Nakata, Takahashi, Ikeda, Haratani, Hojou, and Araki (2007), who reported an association between conflict and sleep-related breathing disturbances known to be a significant determinant of accidents on the job.

Withdrawal from work can take the form of both mental (i.e., daydreaming) and physical (i.e., turnover, absenteeism) escape behaviors. This form of behavioral strain has been found to relate to both interpersonal and intragroup conflict in organizations. According to Spector et al. (2006), these behavioral strains serve the functional purpose of avoiding the stressful or threatening situation at work. Studies using a checklist of withdrawal behaviors indicate a modest positive correlation with interpersonal conflict (Bruk-Lee, Nixon, & Spector, submitted; Spector et al., 2006). Turnover intentions, assessed as a predictor of subsequent turnover, and absenteeism are also greater among employees reporting more conflict with others at work (i.e., clients, peers, or supervisors) or in their work teams (Frone, 2000; Giebels & Janssen, 2005; Harris, Harvey, & Kacmar, 2009; Jehn, 1995; Rainey, 1995).

Another stream of research has cited counterproductive work behaviors (CWB) as a common behavioral reaction to interpersonal conflict in the workplace. These behaviors by employees are aimed at hurting the organization and/or the individuals who are a part of it. We include CWBs as relevant to well-being given that aggression and hostility can cause harm to others, in addition to the self. Studies indicate that employees who report more relationship-based conflict at work engage in CWBs aimed at both the organization and its members (Bruk-Lee & Spector, 2006; Fox, Spector, Goh, & Bruursema, 2001). In particular, conflict has been associated with interpersonal aggression, sabotage, and hostility (Chen & Spector, 1992). These relationships were also found when examining cross-source data (self- and peer reports), thus providing evidence for the robustness of the relationship (Fox et al., 2007).

A CONTINGENCY VIEW OF THE CONFLICT-STRAIN RELATIONSHIP

We have presented a stress-based perspective of conflict at work that has been predominantly influenced by an empirical inquiry to understand the strains associated with experiencing dysfunctional or negative encounters with others in the workplace. From this perspective, it may be posited that the emergence of conflict is almost always associated with detriments to well-being. However, to say that conflict cannot play a positive role in organizations would challenges decades of research focused on organizational outcomes of productivity, creativity, and idea generation (see Amason, 1996; Baron, 1991; Fiol, 1994; Tjosvold et al., 1992). Instead, researchers have raised the importance of moderating variables in affecting the potential outcomes of conflict incidents (De Dreu et al., 2004). For example, De Dreu, Harinck, and Van Vianen (1999) proposed four factors—conflict experience, conflict management, conflict results, and types of conflict—as potential influences over conflict outcomes.

The model presented acknowledges the importance of moderator variables at various points in the social stress process. By doing so, we support the need to extend research beyond taxonomy-based studies. That is, while there is significant value in understanding the differential effects of conflict types on employee well-being given the scarcity of research using non-relationship-based conflict measures, it is also necessary to investigate the contingencies that may come into play to impact key outcomes. A more concerted effort to investigate moderator variables in relation to performance-related outcomes can be found in the literature; however, their inclusion in studies of employee psychological and physical health is more limited. This is not surprising considering that the conceptualization of conflict as a social stressor relevant to well-being has evolved over the past decade, with a growing body of research being published in just the last several years.

Nonetheless, a variety of moderator variables have been included in studies measuring well-being criteria, such as conflict management styles (Dijkstra, De Dreu, Evers, & Van Dierendonck, 2009), third-party help (Giebels & Janssen, 2005), organizational culture (Guerra et al., 2005), organizational commitment (Lu, Siu, & Lu, 2010), social support (Thomas, Bliese, & Jex, 2005), job characteristics (Matthews et al., 2000), and personality (Heinisch & Jex, 1997). We present a brief overview of the findings related to conflict management styles and personality given that these have received the greatest attention and are, thus, included in our model.

Personality and the Social Stressor Process

The social stressor model proposes an interaction between aspects of the situation and one's personal tendencies which may shape perceptions and impact outcomes. Trait anxiety, negative affectivity (NA), trait anger, locus of control, Type A, and the five-factor model, to a lesser extent, have all been examined in relation to conflict at work.

Negative affectivity refers to a tendency for experiencing negative emotions and dissatisfaction across situations and time (Watson & Clark, 1984). Individuals who are high on NA will tend to experience frequent anxiety and other negative emotions. While only a limited number of strains have been examined, support for significant moderation has been reported in the relation of conflict to CWBs (Bowling & Eschlman, 2010; Penney & Spector, 2005), depression (Heinisch & Jex, 1997), and overall negative mood (Bolger & Zuckerman, 1995). In other words, individuals high on NA tend to respond more than individuals low in NA to conflict with strains. An additional set of studies has reported a positive direct relationship between NA and interpersonal conflict at work (Chen & Spector, 1991; Spector & Jex, 1998; Spector & O'Connell, 1994), suggesting that those high in the trait may be more sensitive to their environment and, hence, perceive more conflict. Similar conclusions have been made regarding trait anxiety (Fox, Spector, & Miles, 2001), defined as the tendency to perceive situations as threatening, and trait anger (Fox & Spector, 1999; Fox et al., 2001), defined as the propensity to perceive situations to be anger provoking (Spielberger, 1979). As with trait anger, the impatience/irritability component of the Type A personality, which refers to one's tendency to experience anger and frustration, has been found to have a positive correlation with conflict in studies with longitudinal designs (Spector & O'Connell, 1994).

Locus of control (LOC) refers to a generalized belief that either one's actions or external forces control outcomes and rewards (Rotter, 1966). Typically, individuals who believe that they are in control are referred to as "internal," while those who believe they lack control are labeled "external." Locus of control has been studied in relation to various spheres, including the workplace and interpersonal relationships (Paulhus, 1983; Spector, 1982). The few studies investigating the role of LOC in the conflict process have been contradictory. On the one hand, it has been suggested that externals would evaluate conflict situations as being more stressful due to their lack of control over the social environment. Longitudinal support for this view found that externals report more conflict than internals over time (Spector & O'Connell, 1994). However, Hahn (2000) reported stronger conflict–strain relationships for internals and suggested that this may be due to incongruence between perceived and actual control. This is particularly relevant to social stressors in which the conflict situation may be initiated by someone else and one may have little control over another's actions.

The Five Factor Model (FFM, Digman, 1990) of personality is a widely accepted framework of personality made up of five broad dimensions, including agreeableness, openness, conscientiousness, extraversion, and neuroticism (Barrick & Mount, 1991). Of these, agreeableness, which refers to a tendency for being flexible, forgiving, cooperative, good-natured, trusting, and helpful, as well as conscientiousness, defined as tendency to be organized, self-disciplined, punctual, careful, and responsible, have received some attention in relation to conflict in the workplace. Not surprisingly, studies have shown that individuals rated high in agreeableness display fewer conflict-provoking behaviors (Venkataramani & Dalal, 2007). Jockin, Arvey, and McGue (2001) reported that individuals lower in the personality dimension of control, which was used in their study as a proxy measure for conscientiousness, engaged in more workplace aggression and conflict.

Conflict Management Styles and the Social Stressor Process

In addition to personality differences, individuals differ in the way in which they manage incidents of conflict at work. The goal of conflict management is to maximize the constructive aspects of conflict and minimize its detrimental outcomes, including those related to well-being. Conflict management styles can vary across situations and are influenced by previous success using a specific style, the style of the other party involved, and specific norms surrounding conflict situations (Bruk-Lee, 2006). Various models of conflict management styles ranging from two to five styles have received support and attention (see Deutsch, 1949; Rahim, 2001). Conflict styles are typically categorized into two dimensions, including concern for self and concern for others. Different styles of conflict management fall at various points along these two dimensions and, hence, will be chosen based on an individual's preferences. The more inclusive and commonly studied conflict styles include avoiding, obliging, dominating, integrating, and compromising (see Rahim, 2001).

As with other moderators, very few studies have tested the impact of various conflict management styles in relation to employee well-being. Dijkstra et al. (2009) recently studied the use of four different conflict styles across three separate samples. The researchers concluded that individuals who engaged in passive conflict styles, including avoiding and yielding, experienced more strains in response to conflict situations at work. Similarly, Van Dierendonck and Mevissen (2002) suggested that the use of avoiding and yielding conflict styles could result in increased frustration and, hence, negatively impact health. In fact, a study by De Dreu, Van Dierendonck, and de Best-Waldhober (2002) reported higher levels of somatic complaints for individuals using avoiding, yielding, and forcing conflict styles in response to interpersonal conflict. In turn, integrating and compromising conflict styles have been found to buffer the conflict-strain relationship up to a certain point beyond which using these styles can also be linked to increased strain (Chung-Yan & Moeller, 2010). An alternate view suggests that an individual's chosen conflict style influences the environment around them in such a ways that they encounter more or less stress. For example, Friedman, Tidd, Currall, and Tsai (2000) reported that employees who engaged in integrative conflict styles experienced lower levels of task conflict, which were associated with reduced experiences of relationship conflict and, consequently, strains.

PRACTICAL IMPLICATIONS AND CONCLUDING REMARKS

Social interactions with customers, patients, peers, and supervisors play an important role in today's rapidly changing workplace. The opportunity for workplace conflict, whether task- or relationship-based, is present on a daily basis. Over time, we have trained managers to consider task-based conflicts as positive forces that can stimulate creativity and generate quality ideas. However, we are more recently discovering that conflict, regardless of its potential organizational benefits, is generally associated with detriments to employee well-being. How, then, do we reconcile these two findings to promote conflict while safeguarding the health of our employees?

Recent studies have attempted to find a concise answer to this question. While we are still in the early stages of understanding the conflict–well-being connection, we can derive practical recommendations. Equipping employees with useful ways to identify the emergence of conflict and effective techniques for managing and resolving these incidents can reduce the severity of strains experienced. For example, employees can be trained in the behaviors associated with each conflict style and given recommendations on when and how to apply them. Removing or addressing organizational barriers that are commonly linked to conflict, such as organizational constraints and ambiguous assignments, can also help reduce the negative impact on employee well-being. Training employees on ways in which to stop the conflict spiral, so that they are able to recognize and stop task-based conflicts from turning personal also merits consideration. Specifically, increasing team cohesiveness and trust among employees is one approach expected to reduce the conflict spiral given that employees would be less likely to misattribute the intentions behind a task-based conflict as being personally driven. Cohesiveness and trust can be enhanced through the use of team-building efforts by management through both formal team-building training programs and management actions. The former consists of team experiences with a trainer who conducts exercises that can enhance team communication skills and a sense of teamwork. The latter can be performed by managers who assign challenging tasks to groups that need cooperation rather than competition for successful completion, and who pay close attention to interactions among subordinates in order to intervene when necessary to resolve emerging conflicts. Investing in stress management programs can also give employees useful tools for coping with their emotions before they manifest as further strains, such as withdrawal.

With increased globalization, employers are also experiencing growing diversity in their workforces. While the impact of diversity on conflict's work-related outcomes (e.g., performance and commitment) has received some attention (see Jehn, Chadwick, & Thatcher, 1997; Jehn, Northcraft, & Neale, 1999; Pelled, Eisenhardt, & Xin, 1999), its influence on the conflict–well-being link remains largely unexplored. Findings suggest that diversity with regards to work-related values, gender, and age predicts the occurrence of relationship conflict within work groups and, in some cases, reduced satisfaction (Jehn et al., 1999). Nevertheless, it is important to note that some forms of diversity (i.e., social category diversity) within groups may increase the likelihood of positive outcomes, such as group morale (see Jehn et al., 1999). From a practical perspective, this suggests that diversity awareness training as well as careful consideration of workforce composition have potential for mitigating conflict in an ever-changing workplace.

The social work environment can be a source of satisfaction, enabling the formation of meaningful relationships with others. It can also lead to the experience of disagreements and heated disputes that may be accompanied by a variety of negative emotions and strains. A stress framework is a useful way to conceptualize conflict as a leading workplace stressor. Additional studies are needed to further clarify the conflict–well-being connection and understand the contingencies that affect this relationship. We hope that with increased attention to this area of study will come further recommendations for practice.

REFERENCES

Abrahamson, K., Anderson, J.G., Anderson, M.M., Suitor, J.J., & Pillemer, K. (2010). The cumulative influence of conflict on nursing home staff. *Research in Gerontology Nursing. 3*, 39–48.

Amason, A.C. (1996). Distinguishing the effects of functional and dysfunctional conflict on strategic decision making: Resolving a paradox for top management teams. *Academy of Management Journal, 39*, 123–148.

Amason, A.C., & Schweiger, D.M. (1994). Resolving the paradox of conflict, strategic decision making, and organizational performance. *International Journal of Conflict Management, 5,* 239–253.

American Heart Association. (2010). *Stress and heart disease.* Retrieved from http://www.americanheart.org.

Appelberg, K., Romanov, K., Heikkila, K., Honkasalo, M.L., & Koskenvuo, M. (1996). Interpersonal conflict as a predictor of work disability: A follow-up study of 15,348 Finnish employees. *Journal of Psychosomatic Research, 40,* 157–167.

Appelberg, K., Romanov, K., Honkasalo, M.L., & Koskenvuo, M. (1991). Interpersonal Conflict at work and psychological characteristics of employees. *Social Science Medicine, 32,* 1051–1056.

Barki, H., & Hartwick, J. (2001). Interpersonal conflict and its management in information systems development. *MIS Quaterly, 25,* 217–250.

Barki, H., & Hartwick, J. (2004). Conceptualizing The Construct of Interpersonal Conflict. *International Journal of Conflict Management, 15,* 216–244.

Baron, R.A. (1991). Positive effects of conflict: A cognitive perspective. *Employee Responsibilities and Rights Journal, 2,* 25–36.

Barrick, M. R., & Mount, M. K. (1991). The big five personality dimensions and job performance: A meta-analysis. *Personnel Psychology, 44,* 1–26.

Bolger, N., DeLongis, A., Kessler, R.C., & Schilling, E.A. (1989). Effects of daily stress on negative mood. *Journal of Personality and Social Psychology, 57,* 808–818.

Bolger, N., & Zuckerman, A. (1995). A frame work for studying personality in the stress process. *Journal of Personality and Social Psychology, 57,* 808–818.

Bowling, N. A., & Beehr, T. A. (2006). Workplace harassment from the victim's perspective: A theoretical model and meta-analysis. *Journal of Applied Psychology, 91,* 998–1012.

Bowling, N. A., & Eschleman, K. J. (2010). Employee personality as a moderator of the relationships between work stressors and counterproductive work behavior. *Journal of Occupational Health Psychology, 15*(1), 91–103.

Brondolo, E., Karlin, W., Alexander, K., Bobrow, A., & Schwartz, J. (1999). Workday communication and ambulatory blood pressure: Implications for the reactivity hypothesis. *Psychophysiology, 36*(1), 86–94.

Bruk-Lee, V. (2006). *Measuring social stressors in organizations: The development of the Interpersonal Conflict in Organizations Scale (ICOS).* (Doctoral dissertation, University of South Florida). Available from ProQuest Dissertations & Theses database. (UMI No. 3248288)

Bruk-Lee, V., Nixon, A.E., & Spector, P.E. (submitted). *Conflict at work and employee well-being: Good for business? Not for me.* Manuscript submitted for publication.

Bruk-Lee, V., & Spector, P.E. (2006). The social stressors–counterproductive work behaviors link: Are conflicts with supervisors and coworkers the same? *Journal of Occupational Health Psychology, 11,* 145–156.

Chen, P. Y., & Spector, P. E. (1991). Negative affectivity as the underlying cause of correlations between stressors and strains. *Journal of Applied Social Psychology, 30,* 867–885.

Chen, P.Y., & Spector, P.E. (1992). Relationships of work stressors with aggression, withdrawal, theft and substance use: An exploratory study. *Journal of Occupational and Organizational Psychology, 65,* 177–184.

Chung-Yan, G.A., & Moeller, C. (2010). The psychosocial costs of conflict management styles. *International Journal of Conflict Management, 21,* 382–399.

De Dreu, C.K.W. (2008). The virtue and vice of workplace conflict: Food for (pessimistic) thought. *Journal of Organizational Behavior, 29,* 5–18.

De Dreu, C.K.W., & Gelfand, M.J. (Eds.). (2007). *The psychology of conflict and conflict management in organizations.* SIOP Organizational Frontiers Series. Mahwah, NJ: Erlbaum.

De Dreu, C.K.W., Harinck, F., & Van Vianen, A.E.M. (1999). Conflict and performance in groups and organizations. In C.L.Cooper & I. Robertson (Eds.), *International review of industrial and organizational psychology* (Vol.14, pp. 369–414). Chichester, UK: Wiley.

De Dreu, C.K.W., Van Dierendonck, D., & De Best-Waldhober, M. (2002). Conflict at work and individual well-being. In M. Schabracq, J.A.M. Winnubst, & C.L. Cooper (Eds.), *International handbook of work and health psychology* (pp. 495–626). Chichester, UK: Wiley.

De Dreu, C.K.W., Van Dierendonck, D., & Dijkstra, M. (2004). Conflict at work and individual well-being. *International Journal of Conflict Management, 15,* 6–26.

De Dreu, C.K.W., & Weingart, L.R. (2003). Task versus relationship conflict, team performance, and team member satisfaction: A meta-analysis. *Journal of Applied Psychology, 88,* 741–749.

Deutsch, M. (1949). A theory of cooperation and competition. *Human Relations, 2,* 129–151.

Digman, J. M. (1990). Personality structure: Emergence of the five-factor model. *Annual Review of Psychology, 41,* 417–440.

Dijkstra, M. T. M., De Dreu, C. K. W., Evers, A., & Van Dierendonck, D. (2009). Passive responses to interpersonal conflict at work amplify employee strain. *European Journal of Work and Organizational Psychology, 18*(4), 405–423.

Dormann, C., & Zapf, D. (1999). Social support, social stressors at work, and depressive symptoms: Testing for main and moderating effects with structural equations in a three-wave longitudinal study. *Journal of Applied Psychology, 84,* 874–884.

Dormann, C., & Zapf, D. (2002). Social stressors at work, irritation, and depressive symptoms: Accounting for unmeasured third variables in a multi-wave study. *Journal of Occupational and Organizational Psychology, 75,* 33–58.

Fiol, C.M. (1994). Consensus, diversity and learning in organizations. *Organization Science, 5,* 403–420.

Fox, S., & Spector, P. E. (1999). A model of work frustration-aggression. *Journal of Organizational Behavior, 20,* 915–931.

Fox, S., Spector, P. E., Goh, A., & Bruursema, K. (2007). Does your coworker know what you're doing? Convergence of self- and peer-reports of counterproductive work behavior. *International Journal of Stress Management, 14,* 41–60.

Fox, S., Spector, P.E., & Miles, D. (2001). Counterproductive work behavior (CWB) in response to job stressors and organizational justice: Some mediator and moderator tests for autonomy and emotions. *Journal of Vocational Behavior, 59,* 1–19.

Friedman, R.A., Tidd, S.T., Currall, S.C., & Tsai, J.C. (2000). What goes around comes around: The impact of personal conflict style on work conflict and stress. *The International Journal of Conflict Management, 11,* 32–55.

Frone, M.R. (1998). Predictors of work injuries among employed adolescents. *Journal of Applied Psychology, 83,* 565–576.

Frone, M.R. (2000). Interpersonal conflict at work and psychological outcomes: Testing a model among young workers. *Journal of Occupational Health Psychology, 5,* 246–255.

Giebels, E., & Janssen, O. (2005). Conflict stress and reduced well-being at work: The buffering effect of third-party help. *European Journal of Work and Organizational Psychology, 14*(2), 137–155.

Guerra, J. M., Martinez, I., Munduate, L., & Medina, F. J. (2005). A contingency perspective on the study of the consequences of conflict types: The role of organizational culture. *European Journal of Work and Organizational Psychology, 14*(2), 157–176.

Hahn, S.E. (2000). The effects of locus of control on daily exposure, coping and reactivity to work interpersonal stressors: A diary study. *Personality and Individual Differences, 29,* 729–748.

Harris, K. J., Harvey, P., & Kacmar, K. M. (2009). Do social stressors impact everyone equally? An examination of the moderating impact of core self-evaluations. *Journal of Business & Psychology, 24*(2), 153–164.

Haug, T.T., Mykletum, A., & Dahl, A.A. (2004). The association between anxiety, depression, and somatic symptoms in a large population: The HUNT-II Study. *Psychosomatic Medicine, 66,* 845–851.

Heinisch, D.A., & Jex, S.M. (1997). Negative affectivity and gender as moderators of the relationship between work-related stressors and depressed mood at work. *Work and Stress, 11,* 46–57.

Hemingway, M.A., & Smith, C.S. (1999). Organizational climate and occupational stressors as predictors of withdrawal behaviours and injuries in nurses. *Journal of Occupational and Organizational Psychology, 72,* 285–299.

Hershcovis, M. S. (In press). "Incivility, social undermining, bullying… oh my!" A call to reconcile constructs within workplace aggression research. *Journal of Organizational Behavior.*

Inoue, A., & Kawakami, N. (2010). Interpersonal conflict and depression among Japanese workers with high or low socioeconomic status: Findings from the Japan Work Stress and Health Cohort Study. *Social Science & Medicine, 71,* 173–180.

Jehn, K.A. (1994). Enhancing effectiveness: An investigation of advantages and disadvantages of value-based intragroup conflict. *International Journal of Conflict Management, 5,* 223–238.

Jehn, K.A. (1995). A multimethod examination of the benefits and detriments of intragroup conflict. *Administrative Science Quarterly, 40,* 256–282.

Jehn, K.A. (1997). A qualitative analysis of conflict types and dimensions in organizational groups. *Administrative Science Quarterly, 42,* 530–557.

Jehn, K.A., Northcraft, G.B., & Neale, M.A. (1999). Why differences make a difference: A field study of diversity, conflict, and performance in workgroups. *Administrative Science Quarterly, 44,* 741–763.

Jehn, K.A., Chadwick, C., & Thatcher, S. (1997). To agree or not to agree: The effects of value congruence, individual demographic dissimilarity, and conflict on workgroup outcomes. *International Journal of Conflict Management, 8*, 287–305.

Jockin, V., Arvey, R.D., & McGue, M. (2001). Perceived victimization moderates self-reports of workplace aggression and conflict. *Journal of Applied Psychology, 86*, 1262–1269.

Johnston, J.J. (1995). Occupational injury and stress. *Journal of Occupational and Environmental Medicine*, 37, 199–203.

Lavoie, K.L., Miller, S.B., Conway, M., & Fleet, R.P. (2001). Anger, negative emotions, and cardiovascular reactivity during interpersonal conflict in women. *Journal of Psychosomatic Research, 51*, 503–512.

Lazarus, R.S. (1999). *Stress and emotion: A new synthesis.* New York, NY: Springer.

Lazuras, L., Rodafinos, A., Matsiggos, G., & Stamatoulakis, A. (2009). Perceived occupational stress, affective, and physical well-being among telecommunication employees in Greece. *Social Science & Medicine, 68*, 1075–1081.

Liu, C., Spector, P. E., & Shi, L. (2007). Cross-national job stress: A quantitative and qualitative study. *Journal of Organizational Behavior, 28*, 209–239.

Lu, L., Siu, O.L., & Lu, C.Q. (2010). Does loyalty protect Chinese workers from stress? The role of affective organizational commitment in the Greater China region. *Stress and Health, 26*, 161–168.

Macdonald, S. (1995). The role of drugs in workplace injuries: Is drug testing appropriate? *Journal of Drug Issues, 25*, 703–722.

Maslach, C. (1982). *Burnout: The cost of caring.* Englewood Cliffs, NJ: Prentice Hall.

Matthews, K. A., Raikkonen, K., Everson, S. A., Flory, J. D., Marco, C. A., Owens, J. F., & Lloyd, C. E. (2000). Do the daily experiences of healthy men and women vary according to occupational prestige and work strain? *Psychosomatic Medicine, 62*(3), 346–353.

Nakata, A., Takahashi, M., Ikeda, T., Haratani, T., Hojou, M., & Araki, S. (2007). Perceived job stress and sleep-related breathing disturbance in Japanese male workers. *Social Science & Medicine, 64*, 2520–2532.

Narayanan, L., Menon, S., & Spector, P.E. (1999a). A cross-cultural comparison of job stressors and reaction among employees holding comparable jobs in two countries. *International Journal of Stress Management, 6*, 197–212.

Narayanan, L., Menon, S., & Spector, P.E. (1999b). Stress in the workplace: A comparison of gender and occupations. *Journal of Organizational Behavior, 20*, 63–73.

Nixon, A. E., Mazzola, J. J., Bauer, J., Krueger, J. R., & Spector, P. E. (2011). Can work make you sick? A meta-analysis of the relationships between job stressors and physical symptoms. *Work & Stress, 25*, 1–22.

Paulhus, D. (1983). Sphere-specific measures of perceived control. *Journal of Personality and Social Psychology, 44*, 1253–1265.

Pearson, C.M., Andersson, L.M., & Porath, C.L. (2005). Workplace incivility. In S. Fox & P. E. Spector (Eds.), *Counterproductive work behavior: Investigations of actors and targets* (pp. 177–200). Washington, DC: American Psychological Association.

Pelled, L.H., Eisenhardt, K.M., & Xin, K.R. (1999). Exploring the black box: An analysis of work group diversity, conflict, and performance. *Administrative Science Quarterly, 44,* 1–28.

Penney, L. M., & Spector, P. E. (2005). Job stress, incivility, and counterproductive work behavior (CWB): The moderating role of negative affectivity. *Journal of Organizational Behavior, 26*(7), 777–796.

Piferi, R.L., & Lawler, K.A. (2000). Hostility and the cardiovascular reactivity of women during interpersonal confrontation. *Women & Health, 30,* 111–129.

Pinkley, R.L. (1990). Dimensions of conflict frame: Disputant interpretations of conflict. *Journal of Applied Psychology, 75,* 117–126.

Rahim, M. A. (2001). *Managing conflict in organizations* (3rd ed.). Westport, CT: Quorum.

Rainey, D.W. (1995). Sources of stress among baseball and softball umpires. *Journal of Applied Sport Psychology, 7,* 1–10.

Rayner, C., & Keashly, L. (2005). Bullying at work: A perspective from Britain and North America. In S. Fox & P. E. Spector (Eds.), *Counterproductive work behavior: Investigations of actors and targets.* (pp. 271–296). Washington, DC: American Psychological Association.

Rotter, J. B. (1966). Generalized expectations for internal versus external control of reinforcement. *Psychological Monographs, 80*(1), 1–28.

Schnall, P.L, Schwartz, J.E., Landsbergis, P.A., Warren, K., & Pickering, T.G. (1998). A longitudinal study of job strain and ambulatory blood pressure: Results from a three-year follow-up. *Psychosomatic Medicine, 60,* 697–706.

Shaw, L., & Sichel, H. S. (1971). *Accident proneness.* Oxford, England: Pergamon Press.

Shirom, A., Westman, M., Shamai, O., & Carel, R. S. (1997). Effects of work overload and burnout on cholesterol and triglycerides levels: The moderating effects of emotional reactivity among male and female employees. *Journal of Occupational Health Psychology, 2,* 275–288.

Simons, T.L., & Peterson, R.S. (2000). Task conflict and relationship conflict in top management teams: The pivotal role of intragroup trust. *Journal of Applied Psychology, 85,* 102–111.

Smith, M., Cohen, H.H., Cohen, A., & Cleveland, R. (1978). Characteristics of successful safety programs. *Journal of Safety Research, 10,* 5–15.

Smith, M.J., Karsh, B.T., Carayon, P., & Conway, F.T. (2003). Controlling occupational safety and health hazards. In J.C. Quick & L.E. Tetrick (Eds.). *Handbook of occupational health psychology* (pp. 35–68). Washington, DC: American Psychological Association.

Spector, P. E. (1982). Behavior in organizations as a function of employee's locus of control. *Psychological Bulletin, 91,* 482–497.

Spector, P. E., & Bruk-Lee, V. (2008). Conflict, health, and well-being. In C. K. W. De Dreu & M. J. Gelfand (Eds.), *The psychology of conflict and conflict management in organizations* (pp. 267–288). San Francisco, CA: Jossey-Bass.

Spector, P. E., Coulter, M. L., Stockwell, H. G., & Matz, M. W. (2007). Perceived violence climate: A new construct and its relationship to workplace physical violence and verbal aggression, and their potential consequences. *Work & Stress, 21,* 117–130.

Spector, P. E., Fox, S., Penney, L. M., Bruursema, K., Goh, A., & Kessler, S. (2006). The dimensionality of counterproductivity: Are all counterproductive behaviors created equal? *Journal of Vocational Behavior, 68,* 446–460.

Spector, P.E., & Jex, S.M. (1998). Development of four self-report measures of job stressors and strain: Interpersonal Conflict at Work Scale, Organizational Constraint Scale, Quantitative Workload Inventory, and Physical Symptoms Inventory. *Journal of Occupational Health Psychology, 3,* 356–367.

Spector, P.E., & O'Connell, B.J. (1994). The contribution of personality traits, negative affectivity, locus of control and Type A to the subsequent reports of job stressors and job strains. *Journal of Occupational and Organizational Psychology, 67,* 1–11.

Spielberger, C. D. (1979). *Preliminary manual for the state-trait personality inventory (STPI).* University of South Florida, Tampa.

Thomas, J. L., Bliese, P. D., & Jex, S., M. (2005). Interpersonal conflict and organizational commitment: Examining two levels of supervisory support as multilevel moderators. *Journal of Applied Psychology, 35*(11), 2375–2398.

Tidd, S.T., McIntyre, H.H., & Friedman, R.A. (2004). The importance of role ambiguity and trust in conflict perception: Unpacking the task conflict to relationships conflict linkage. *International Journal of Conflict Management, 15,* 364–380.

Tjosvold, D., Dann, V., & Wong, C. (1992). Managing conflict between departments to serve customers. *Human Relations, 4,* 1035–1054.

Van Dierendonck, D., & Mevissen, N. (2002). Aggressive behavior of passengers, conflict management behavior, and burnout among trolley car drivers. *International Journal of Stress Management, 9,* 345–356.

Van Dijkhuizen, N., & Reiche, H. (1980). Psychosocial stress in industry: A heartache for middle management? *Psychotherapy and psychosomatics, 34,* 124–134.

Venkataramani, V., & Dalal, R.S. (2007). Who helps and harms whom? Relational antecedents of interpersonal helping and harming in organizations. *Journal of Applied Psychology, 92,* 952–966.

Watson, D., & Clark, L.A. (1984). Negative affectivity: The disposition to experience aversive emotional states. *Psychological Bulletin, 96,* 495–490.

CHAPTER 2

ORGANIZATIONAL IDENTITY, SOCIAL SUPPORT SYSTEMS, AND OCCUPATIONAL STRESS

The Development of a Conceptual Model

Jason Stoner
Ohio University

Pamela L. Perrewé
Florida State University

ABSTRACT

A theoretical model is developed to illustrate the role of identity and identity hierarchies in the organizational stress process. Using the dimensions and the strength of the dimensions of identity, we explain how identities are arranged in a hierarchy and how identity influences perceptions of organizational situations. Furthermore, we explain how identity hierarchies affect how employees perceive organizational stressors and the use of social support systems. Finally, we propose that identity hierarchies will be readjusted based on the effectiveness of social support systems. Testable propositions are provided, as are implications for practice.

Coping and Prevention, pages 23–41

Identity, or how individuals define themselves in relation to the various social groups with which they interact, serves as a perceptual lens through which individuals view the world (e.g., Stryker & Burke, 2000; Stryker & Serpe, 1982). Recently, identity has received much research attention in the organizational sciences. In this chapter, we examine how individuals' identities become more or less salient in the context of identity hierarchies, as well as the role of identity in the stress and coping process. For example, employees who identify strongly with their work or career may experience more anxiety than employees who do not identify with their work, when faced with a stressor in the workplace. Thus, the strength of identities has strong implications regarding employee attitudes and behaviors.

This chapter extends the identity research in several ways. First, we argue that the dimensions constituting identity can be used to determine identity and social support hierarchies. Second, we argue that identity hierarchies facilitate information processing such that workplace stimuli that threaten identities higher in one's identity hierarchy are more likely to be viewed as stressors. Furthermore, we posit that social support systems higher in one's social support hierarchy will be used in attempts to mitigate felt strain. Finally, we conclude that the effectiveness of individuals' social support systems will influence the strength of the dimensions that constitute identity. In doing so, we develop a theoretical model (see Figure 2.1) that provides specific propositions illustrating the interplay of identity, social support, and stress. We examine the conceptual background supporting our model and then examine the detail of the model later in this chapter. Finally, we highlight the research and management implications of the proposed model.

CURRENT STATE OF THE IDENTITY LITERATURE

In this section, research on identity and stress is reviewed. First, the origins of social identity are delineated, followed by a review of identity salience. Next, identity is defined, with particular emphasis placed on the dimensionality of identity (e.g., Ashmore, Deaux, & McLaughlin-Volpe, 2004). Organizational identity and identities outside the organization are discussed, and the current use of identity in the organizational sciences is reviewed, highlighting the limitations of current research.

The Roots of Social Identity

"Who am I?" is a question that individuals have long asked themselves (e.g., Mead, 1934). One way to conceptualize oneself is in relation to society or social groups, known as social identity. Social identity can be concep-

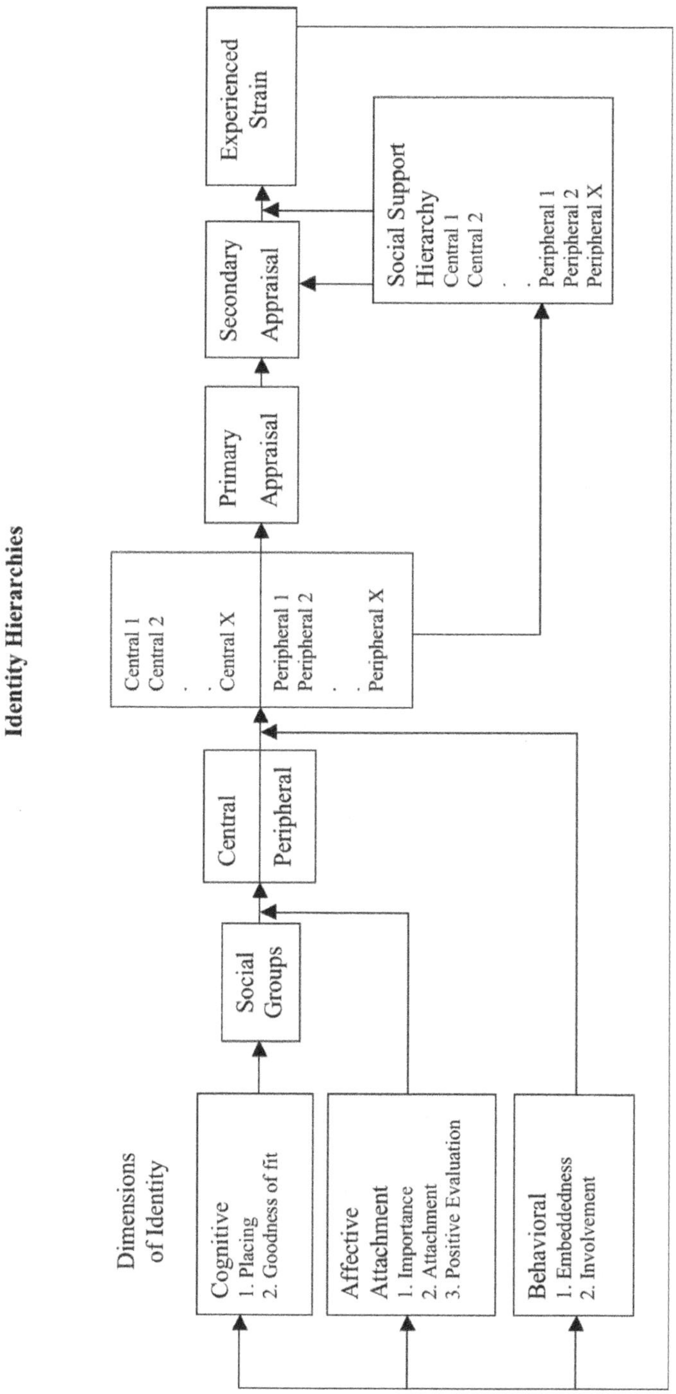

Figure 2.1 The role of identity in the organizational stress process.

tualized as an "individual's knowledge that he belongs to a certain group together with some emotional and value significance to him of this group" (Tajfel, 1972, p. 292). As noted by Hogg and Terry (2001), a system of social categorizations helps create and define "an individual's own place in society" (Tajfel, 1972, p. 293). Social identity theory's basic premise is that the social categories into which one falls, and to which one feels attached, provide "a definition of who one is in terms of defining characteristics of the category—a self-definition that is part of the self-concept" (Hogg & Terry, 2001, p. 3).

Individuals hold many identities at once, which are cognitively arranged in a hierarchy according to some sort of subjective importance (Ashforth, 2001; Kreiner, Hollensbe, & Sheep, 2006). Based on the work of cognitive social psychologists (e.g., Markus, 1977), identity researchers have suggested that identities that are more salient (i.e., higher in the cognitive hierarchy) will have a higher probability of being invoked across a variety of situations (Stryker & Burke, 2000). Identities that are salient drive cognitive interpretations of situations, and thus influence behavior (Stryker & Burke, 2000).

Which Social Identity Is Salient?

The identity that emerges and guides behavior generally is based on two factors. First, individuals have a tendency to cognitively match aspects, or characteristics, of social groups to the situational context. For instance, McCall and Simmons (1978) noted that one hierarchy that individuals cognitively hold is the situational self—a hierarchy that ranks identities in terms of the likelihood that adopting such an identity will result in positive outcomes given the social situation. McCall and Simmons' (1978) prominence hierarchy is similar to the concept of social identity hierarchy (e.g., Stryker, 1980), which arranges identities in terms of salience or the likelihood they will be invoked across situations (e.g., Stryker & Serpe, 1994). That is, the second element of identity salience realizes that individuals have an internal preference for one identity over others. An identity that is salient predicts behavior across a variety of situations. For instance, Stryker and Serpe (1994) provided the example of a professor whose salient social identity is teaching, and as such, illustrates this salient identity by lecturing his or her children. We can extend this example to an operations manager who keeps her children on a tight, efficient time schedule for after-school activities.

Dimensions of Identity

Identity researchers (e.g., Ashmore et al., 2004; Deaux, 1996) have long examined the dimensionality of identity, and, discussions of identity dimensions can be conceptually grouped into cognitive, affective, and behavioral categorizations. The components of the cognitive dimension of identity involve both categorizing oneself into a social group and evaluating how well one fits with a social group. The cognitive dimension aligns with the self-categorization dimension of Ashmore et al. (2004). Ashmore and colleagues described self-categorization as the most basic element of identity. Self-categorization refers to simply placing oneself into a specific social group (Deaux, 1996) and goodness-of-fit. Goodness-of-fit pertains to individuals' subjective evaluation of the degree to which they perceive themselves to be similar to the prototypical member of this group (Ashmore et al., 2004).

The affective-attachment dimension encompasses the evaluation and importance of, and the attachment to, a social group. Evaluation refers to "the positive or negative attitude that a person has toward the social category in question" (Ashmore et al., 2004, p. 86). Importance refers to the degree to which a specific group membership has significance to individuals' overall sense of self (Ashmore et al., 2004). Importance is very similar to Stryker and Serpe's (1994, p. 17) concept of salience, which is "a readiness to act out an identity as a consequence of the identity's properties as a cognitive structure or schema," and McCall and Simmon's (1978) term *prominence.* Ashmore et al. (2004, p. 90) described attachment as "the degree to which the fate of the group is perceived as overlapping with one's personal fate."

The behavioral dimension includes social embeddedness and behavioral involvement. Ashmore et al. (2004, p. 92) defined social embeddedness as "the degree to which a particular collective identity is implicated in the person's everyday ongoing social relationships," and this construct refers to individuals' social network and interpersonal relationships. It can range from high to low, depending on the content and context of the majority of individuals' interactions, and there is an understood cost of breaking away from such social roles (Stryker & Serpe, 1994). Ashmore et al. (2004) defined behavioral involvement as the degree to which individuals partake in action based on their identity, and it is a clear expression of the identity itself, that is, the degree to which the individual's behavior represents the group.

Multiple Identities

Ashmore et al. (2004) noted that it is likely that individuals hold several identities at one time. This notion is not novel, as many have suggested identity hierarchies (e.g., Callero, 1985; McCall & Simmons, 1978; Stryker, 1980). That is, the various identities individuals possess are cognitively arranged from most significant to least significant (Stryker, 1980; Stryker & Serpe, 1994).

Foddy and Kashima (2002) distinguished between central and peripheral self-concepts. These researchers contend that central self-concepts are characteristics about which individuals are certain or sure to be defining and enduring characteristics of themselves. Conversely, peripheral self-concepts are characteristics that individuals are less certain represent their true sense of self. Thus, some identities are central identities while some identities are peripheral. We contend that central versus peripheral identities will be arranged differently in the hierarchy in that the former are higher (and the latter are lower) in one's identity hierarchy. However, to date, research has not investigated why some identities are more central, whereas other identities are more peripheral. One of the contributions of this chapter is that we provide theoretical justification for the elements of identity differentially impacting central versus peripheral identities.

Identities Within and Outside the Organization

In recent work on organizational identification, researchers (e.g., Kreiner & Ashforth, 2004) attempted to further our conceptualization of identity in the workplace by more thoroughly examining the ways in which individuals could derive their identity from an organization. These researchers noted that the "organization is merely *one* way that an individual might derive a sense of self" (Kreiner & Ashforth, 2004, p. 2). Identity researchers (e.g., Ashforth & Mael, 1989; Dutton, Dukerich, & Harquail, 1994; Kreiner & Ashforth, 2004) spend considerable time illustrating how identities within the organization (e.g., work group identity versus organizational identity; identification versus misidentification) conflict with each other, and which one prevails as the driving force behind behaviors and attitudes. Research has continued in this realm, for instance, distinguishing between career identity, entrepreneurial identity, job identity, organization identity, and team identity (Washington, 2000). However, these researchers did not extend their research to consider identities that reside outside of the organization and that may conflict with organization and work group identity.

Organizational scientists have begun to examine a select few identities that reside outside of the organization. Research examining diversity in the workplace has noted that a "diversity identity" has organizational implications. For instance, the extent to which women are merely a token in their work setting, rather than a substantial force at work, tends to influence informal interaction patterns (Kanter, 1977). Following Kanter's assertion, Mehra, Kilduff, and Brass (1998) found that a social category is more likely to be the basis for social identification the greater the disparity between that social group and the majority.

Furthermore, Kreiner et al. (2006) empirically examined identity negotiations, noting that individuals consistently struggle between personal identities (e.g., father, husband) and organizational identities. Still, because full-time working individuals spend about 50% of their waking hours outside of work, and the work-force is becoming composed of more and more temporary workers (Segal & Sullivan, 1997), more theoretical and empirical work is needed on the influence of identities that are not work-based.

Consequences of Organizational Identity

Since the late 1960s (e.g., Brown, 1969), organizational identification has been studied as an antecedent to job satisfaction and organizational effectiveness (Ashforth & Mael, 1989). Ashforth and Mael (1989) posited that there are several consequences (e.g., commitment to the organization) of organizational identification that are supported by social identity theory. Further, they argued that organizational identification would be associated with loyalty to and pride in the organization. Ashforth and Mael (1989) asserted that organizational identification would lead to internalization of group values and norms as well as a general homogeneity of attitudes and behaviors.

Dutton and her colleagues (1994) also proposed several consequences of organizational identification. Specifically, their model illustrated a feedback loop that links organizational identification with its antecedents—a reciprocal relationship in which the higher the organizational identity, the more the antecedents will be reinforced. Dutton et al. explained that the greater the organizational identification, the more attractive the members will be to the organization and the more attractive the members will perceive others' perception of the organization. Furthermore, they argued that the stronger the individual's organizational identification, individuals will (1) seek more contact with the organization, (2) have greater cooperation with other organization members, (3) show more competitive behaviors toward out-group members, and (4) more organizational citizenship behaviors will be performed.

In sum, the preponderance of research in the organizational sciences pertaining to identity examines identities in the workplace and the positive consequences of these identities. There has been limited research conducted on (1) the effects of identities that reside outside of the organization, and (2) the possible negative aspects of organizational identity (see van Knippenberg, 2000, for exception). However, one recent study (Das, Dharwadkar, & Brandes, 2008) found that national identity moderated the relationship between organizational identity and performance and stress. Specifically, Das et al. (2008) found that high national identity centrality mitigated that positive effect of organizational identity on performance. Furthermore, these researchers found "that people with high national identity centrality and low OI [organizational identity] experience the highest level of burnout" (Das et al., 2008, p. 1521). Taken together, we develop a theoretical model that examines the role of central identities in the organizational stress process.

The Role of Identity in the Organizational Stress Process

This section proposes a conceptual model of the role of identity in the organizational stress process and offers testable propositions. Specifically, the dimensions of identity are examined as to their effects on four processes. First, we argue that the dimensions of identity differentiate between central and peripheral identities and influence the development of identity hierarchies. Second, we propose that the identity hierarchies will influence which stimuli individuals will perceive as stressors. Third, we propose that identity hierarchies are instrumental in the activation and use of social support. Finally, propositions are offered regarding how the strength of dimensions of identity is influenced by the stress encounter.

Identity theorists (e.g., McCall & Simmons, 1978; Stryker, 1980; Ashforth, 2001) have suggested that individuals have a hierarchy of identities that they cognitively arrange in terms of preference or subjective importance. Das et al. (2008, p. 1501) defined central identity as "the extent to which a person defines himself or herself as a member of a particular social category or the subjective importance of one set of identities (Ashforth, 2001)." Specifically, central identities are identities individuals prefer (i.e., identities that emerge at the top of the identity hierarchy), whereas peripheral identities are the remaining identities individuals possess. A central identity is the identity that emerges if no social cues are present, which would subsequently drive perceptions and behaviors. As depicted in Figure 2.1, we argue that the dimensions of identity can explain how an identity is deemed central versus peripheral and how the dimensions of identity can broaden our understanding of the general organizational stress process.

Central versus Peripheral Identities

Rooted in the works of cognitive psychologists (e.g., Markus, 1977), identity theorists proposed that individuals cognitively arrange identities according to commitment (Stryker & Burke, 2000), based on the number of similar characteristics, or potential positive outcomes associated with a certain identity (e.g., Callero, 1985; McCall & Simmons, 1978; Stryker,

1980). The identity that emerges at the top of the hierarchy is referred to as the central identity.

This is similar to Stryker and Serpe's (1982) term of *salience*. Identities that are more salient are more likely to be evoked in a variety of situations and act as lenses through which individuals interpret situational information, and by which they evaluate appropriate behaviors. Central identities are the identities that individuals prefer and feel most comfortable in and that are a true representation of them. On the other hand, peripheral identities are the remaining identities that individuals possess. Peripheral identities are identities that individuals recognize and activate when deemed necessary. However, individuals do not necessarily prefer these identities, and will try to remain in such roles for limited amounts of time.

The first proposition of the proposed model (see Figure 2.1) concerns the cognitive dimension of identity. In order for a social group to be considered as a central or peripheral identity, individuals must first place themselves in the social group and perceive a good fit with this social group.

> **Proposition 1:** *In order for a social group to be considered an identity, individuals must self-categorize themselves into a social group and perceive a fit with the group.*

In delineating central identities from peripheral identities, we examine three components of the affective attachment dimension of identity. First, an identity must be viewed as important to individuals so that they will internalize it as a central identity. That is, individuals must deem the identity as significant in their life. Likewise, the attachment component plays a role in differentiating between central and peripheral identities. Individuals who view a social group as central to their sense of self and view their fate as the same as that social group will experience a high degree of attachment to that social group (Ashmore et al., 2004). Further, in order for a social group to be considered a central identity, individuals must evaluate the social group positively (Ashmore et al., 2004).

In order for an identity to be internalized as a central identity, individuals must reflect a high degree of attachment and evaluate the group positively. That is, placing a higher degree of importance on an identity and feeling positive and with a high sense of attachment to the social group to which the identity is based will lead to an individual internalizing that identity as truly being a part of him- or herself. Identities, and social groups upon which they are based, that have importance, positive valence, and attachment, will be deemed central identities.

> **Proposition 2:** *Affective-attachment moderates the relationship between social groups to which individuals belong and identity type (i.e., central versus*

peripheral) such that social groups will become central (peripheral) when affective attachment is high (low).

Finally, the behavioral dimension includes social embeddedness and behavioral involvement components. These components are posited to differentiate between numerous central identities and the one central identity that individuals prefer. Drawing from the assertion that individuals hierarchically rank their identities (e.g., Callero, 1985; McCall & Simmons, 1978; Stryker, 1980), it is proposed the degree of social embeddedness and behavioral involvement with each identity will influence the placement of identities. That is, one's salient central identity is the identity that is highest in social embeddedness and behavioral involvement. Furthermore, the remaining central and peripheral identities will be hierarchically arranged according to the degree of social embeddedness and behavioral involvement.

Proposition 3: *Social embeddedness and behavioral involvement moderates the relationship between the numerous central and peripheral identities and the hierarchically arranged central and peripheral identities. Specifically, identities that are higher (lower) in social embeddedness and behavioral involvement will be higher (lower) in the hierarchy, resulting in one salient central identity emerging at the top of the identity hierarchy.*

Identity and Primary Appraisal

Individuals go through a multi-step cognitive process when they encounter potentially threatening stimuli (Lazarus & Folkman, 1987). Models of stress include appraisals of the stimuli and appraisals of the means to cope with the stimuli (Perrewé & Zellars, 1999). The first appraisal, the "primary appraisal," is where individuals first evaluate the stimuli at hand. Here, research has proposed that one of three reactions results in the primary appraisal (Lazarus, 1993). Individuals may dismiss the stimuli as being irrelevant. If this is the case, individuals do not perceive the stimulus as a stressor because the potentially threatening stimulus is seen as unimportant.

Individuals may deem the stimulus as benign or positive. That is, the stimuli are deemed important, but are seen as either not causing harm, or possibly bringing about positive effects. If individuals determine the stimulus as benign or positive in nature, again, no stressor is perceived. However, if individuals perceive a threat as potentially bringing about negative consequences, they will determine the significance of the threat, harm, or challenge. That is, they will determine the degree of harm they will experience from the stressor. If this is high, individuals will experience a greater amount of strain.

Lewin (1936) noted that individuals react to situations based on their perceptions of reality more so than some objective measure of reality.

Along these lines, Lazarus (1993) stressed the importance of individuals' evaluation of stressful situations. Thus, it is likely that identities will influence employees' perceptions of workplace stimuli, thereby influencing the determination of stimuli as threatening or benign. It is proposed that central identities will be more influential in heightening cognitive arousal.

When stimuli are threatening or likely to negatively affect one's salient central identity, those stimuli will be classified as stressors. That is, if a stimulus threatens individuals' ability to act as a prototypical member of their salient central identity, they will feel as though their sense of self is being threatened. Individuals will rank stressors hierarchically according to perceived potential threats to their well-being. Individuals will determine perceived potential threat by how relevant stressors are to one's identity hierarchy. This line of reasoning is consistent with previous research on identity. Specifically, identity theorists have debated the stress-inducing effect of possessing multiple identities (e.g., Clark, Nye & Gecas, 1978; Merton, 1957) versus the stress-mitigating effect of possessing multiple identities (e.g., Verbrugge, 1983). We contend that these philosophical differences lie in the assumption that all identities are created equal. Here, we assert that stimuli that threaten identities that are deemed more important to individuals' sense of self will be more likely to induce strain.

For instance, Bagger, Li and Gutek (2008) found that family interference with work leads to low job satisfaction and high job distress for individuals who do not have a family-based salient identity. As Bagger et al. (2008, p. 190) noted, "when individuals partake in activities that are perceived to affirm one's salient identity, fewer negative outcomes, such as job dissatisfaction and job distress, should result (Crosby, 1991; Epstein, 1987)." Here, we are taking the opposite position with the same perspective. Situations that prohibit individuals from affirming their central identities will be more likely to lead to negative outcomes. It is through appraisal that individuals develop outcome expectations, and expectations determine whether a stimulus becomes a stressor and whether an individual believes that coping is possible. These subjective outcome expectations are fundamental to Cognitive Activation Theory and are the crucial links between potential stressors and the stress experience (Meurs & Perrewé, in press).

Proposition 4: *The higher an identity is in the hierarchy, the more likely threats to that identity will be perceived as a stressor.*

Identity and Secondary Appraisal

During the appraisal, if a stimulus is deemed to be a stressor, individuals will engage in another, secondary appraisal. In this stage, individuals ask themselves if they have the necessary means to deal with the stressor at hand (Folkman & Lazarus, 1985). That is, the secondary appraisal is a cognitive analysis of individuals' belief about their competence of successfully dealing with the stressor (Perrewé & Zellars, 1999). Folkman and Lazarus (1988) asserted that it is the interaction of the stressors at hand with the ability to cope with such stressors that will determine the amount of strain experienced. How effectively an individual is able to cope with stressors is a function of the fit between the stressor and the relevance of the coping mechanism. Social support has been studied from a number of perspectives and is often considered to be one of the most effective methods of coping.

Structural support was deemed similar to possessing a system of supportive others (Cohen & Wills, 1985). Conversely, functional support refers to how individuals use their structural support (Beehr & Glazer, 2001). Beehr and Glazer (2001) suggested that functional support comprised both emotional and instrumental support. Emotional support is reliance on others for interactions that make individuals feel better about themselves (Beehr & Glazer, 2001). Instrumental support refers to tangible supports for helping individuals obtain resources to effectively cope with the stressors (Beehr & Glazer, 2001).

The proposed theoretical model examines the determinants of social support, thus focusing on structural support (i.e., structural support can be functional in that it can be either emotional or instrumental). It is proposed that identities precede social support systems. That is, members of social groups, which constitute identities, act as social supports because individuals will have some social involvement with these members, and place some amount of attachment and importance in the views of other members. In other words, because identities involve categorization with other people into groups that have a good fit, are important, and have some degree of attachment and social involvement, individuals will view such groups as social support systems. Thus, individuals will hold as many social support systems as they do identities. Similar to identity hierarchies, social support groups can be divided into central and peripheral categories.

It is proposed that individuals will cognitively rank their social support systems similarly to their identity hierarchy, and thus, the social support system hierarchy will mirror the identity hierarchy. In other words, social support systems will be higher in one's social support hierarchy when the identity upon which the social support system is based is higher in one's identity hierarchy. As such, individuals will hold one primary central social support system, numerous central social support systems, and numerous peripheral social support systems corresponding to their identity hierarchy.

Proposition 5: *Identities have a corresponding social support system such that the higher the identity in the identity hierarchy, the more likely the corresponding social support system will be high in the social support hierarchy.*

There have been several views as to how social support helps to reduce strain. One hypothesis is that social support systems could be conceptualized as an antecedent to stressors. That is, social support systems are seen as mechanisms for insulating individuals from stressful stimuli, such that individuals with more social support systems do not perceive as many stressors (Viswesvaran, Sanchez, & Fisher, 1999). Subsequently, the more identities individuals possess, the more social support systems they will perceive as being viable options for coping with stressors. Therefore, the greater the number of central identities individuals perceive, the more likely they will feel as though they are able to adequately cope with stressful demands. In sum, during the secondary appraisal, individuals will evaluate their meaning of coping by the number of central social support systems, such that the more central social support systems one perceives, the fewer stressors will be perceived.

Proposition 6: *The more central social support groups individuals perceive, the more likely individuals will perceive they have the means to cope (i.e., secondary appraisal) with a perceived stressor.*

Two other conceptualizations of how social support works to relieve stress are the matching hypothesis (Cohen & Wills, 1985) and the moderating hypothesis (e.g., Ganster, Fusilier, & Mayes, 1986). The matching hypothesis notes that there is a necessary element of matching the aspects of the stressor with an appropriate social support system. That is, having a supportive supervisor may not relieve workplace strain when the supervisor is the stressor (Beehr & Glazer, 2001).

Furthermore, social support can mitigate the negative effects of stressors. For instance, when workplace stressors are high, employees may talk with each other about their discontent, and by venting their frustrations, their negative feelings dissipate. Given these two views of social support, and in the context of the current discussion, one's central social support system will be used to alleviate or reduce the experienced strain.

Proposition 7a: *Individuals will employ their social support hierarchy as a means of coping with stressors.*

Proposition 7b: *Social support centrality will moderate the relationship between secondary appraisal and experienced strain such that the more (less) central the identity, the less (more) experienced strain.*

Experienced Stress and Feedback Loops

After individuals effectively utilize their salient central social support systems to relieve felt strain, individuals will cognitively evaluate why they were able to adequately deal with the stressors. Thus, when strain is not experienced, subconscious and implicit confirmation will be given to their social support hierarchy. They will not see any need to change the hierarchy because the salient central social support system worked as anticipated. In other words, individuals will view their social support hierarchy as adequate. When individuals do not experience strain, they will determine that all appears to be functioning well; thus, they will attempt to maintain their current identity and social support hierarchies.

However, it is possible that the salient central social support system, used in an attempt to reduce experienced strain, may not work. Thus, some individuals will experience strain after they employ their salient central social support system. If individuals do experience strain after the secondary appraisal and the use of their salient central social support system, it is proposed that individuals will reappraise their social support hierarchy by reassessing their salient central identity and the strength of the components of their salient central identity. Lazarus (1993) illustrated a feedback process wherein individuals reevaluate their primary and secondary appraisals based on changes in the coping style and/or the situation. Reappraisal will involve searching for a useful social support system.

Because social support systems are based on identity groups, and central and peripheral identity groups are based on the strength of the dimensions of identity, we argue that ineffective social support groups will be reevaluated as to the strength of their identity dimensions. Specifically, an ineffective social support group will be reevaluated as to placing, goodness of fit, affective attachment, embeddedness, and behavioral involvement. Based on this new assessment, new central identities may emerge, which will lead to new central support groups. Individuals will try several social support groups until they find the one that adequately reduces their experienced strain. At that point, individuals will cognitively adjust their social support hierarchy such that their strain will be relieved by a new salient central social support. In other words, after the old salient central social support system fails, and another support system emerges as relieving their strain based on a new salient central identity, that social support system will now become the salient central support system.

> **Proposition 8:** *Individuals will reassess the strength of the dimensions of identity, their salient central identity, and their salient central social support group after experiencing strain due to an ineffective social support group. The social group associated with the social support most useful in relieving strain will be perceived as having a better fit, higher positive evaluation, importance, attachment, social embeddedness, and behavioral involvement than social groups associated with failed social supports.*

DISCUSSION

This chapter proposes a theoretical model that highlights the relationship between identity and the organizational stress process. Based on various identity theories, the dimensions of collective identity are used to illustrate how individuals cognitively arrange their various identities into their identity hierarchy. Furthermore, the model proposes that the identity hierarchy will influence perceptions of stress, as well as the development and use of social support. Finally, this model proposes that the dimensions of the identity that correspond to effective social support will be reinforced during a cognitive feedback process.

Conceptual and Managerial Contributions

The model proposed extends theory in several ways. Specifically, the proposed model uses the dimensions of identity to explain how identity hierarchies are cognitively arranged. Although previous researchers (e.g., McCall & Simmons, 1978) have examined how identity hierarchies are developed based on various factors such as preference and situational context, there has long been a debate among identity theorists as to what constitutes a "central identity." Some have argued that identities are salient primarily based on contextual congruence. Others have suggested that individuals have one identity that they hold central in almost all occasions. These perspectives are not incompatible, as illustrated in this model. By examining how the dimensions of identity influence identity hierarchies, the model gives credence to both perspectives. That is, the model proposed in this chapter contends that central identities are determined by a combination of identity preference (e.g., self-categorization, attachment) and situational context (e.g., social embeddedness).

Second, our model notes that identity influences perceptions of workplace events. Specifically, stimuli that threaten individuals' central identity will be perceived as stressors. As such, the proposed model addresses the two limits of organizational research pertaining to identity noted earlier in this chapter. That is, the proposed model recognizes that individuals may have a central identity that is based outside of the organization. These individuals are going to be affected by organizational events differently than individuals who have a work-based central identity. For instance, individuals with a family-based central identity will be more likely to experience strain from work–family conflict than individuals with an organization-based central identity. Work–family conflict threatens a family-based central identity by limiting one's ability to act as a prototypical family member. Conversely, work–family conflict is less likely to threaten one's work-based central identity because spending "family time" at work does not limit one's ability to act as a prototypical organizational member.

Further, if an employee has a salient central organization-based identity and views a new promotion policy change (e.g., partner decision made on merit rather than tenure) as potentially threatening her ability to fulfill her organization-based identity (e.g., being a partner in 5 years), she will experience strain. In order to cope with this strain, we contend that she will first turn to others in the organization as a primary support system (e.g., looking to co-workers for emotional support and supervisors for instrumental support). If this support system does not help relieve her strain, she'll turn to other support systems (e.g., family). The identity base that is associated with the support system that finally helps mitigate the strain will become her new salient identity. Over time, her new salient central identity, in our example, will become family-based.

The proposed model also recognizes that organization-based identity may not always be associated with positive outcomes. Specifically, according to the model, individuals with a work-based central identity are going to be bothered more by traditional organizational stressors (e.g., role conflict, psychological contract violation, perceptions of organizational politics) than individuals with a central identity that is not work-based. Because traditional organizational stressors present an obstacle to behaving like a prototypical organizational member, organizational identity is threatened, which causes individuals with a high work-based identity to experience strain. Although this supposition needs to be empirically validated, the proposed model does permit discussion on the possible negative aspects of organizational identity.

Finally, the model proposed in this chapter merges two streams of literature, identity and stress, which contribute to the understanding of how individuals cognitively construct their own reality. Specifically, as Kriener et al. (2006) noted, identity is anything but a static phenomenon, because individuals are constantly reexamining their identities, rather than just once subjectively claiming group membership. Our proposed model notes that identity hierarchies change after stressful events via the individual dimensions of identity. As such, our model provides additional insight into the effects of identity, by presenting a fluid model of identity and stress.

CONCLUSION

This chapter integrates identification and stress research to develop a theoretical model with testable propositions. The model proposes that the dimensions of identity will determine individuals' identity hierarchies. Further, this chapter proposes that individuals' identity hierarchies will influence perceptions of stress, as well as means of coping. Finally, this chapter proposes that identity hierarchies will be revaluated after stressful encounters.

REFERENCES

Ashforth, B.E. (2001). *Role transitions in organizational life: An identity-based perspective.* Mahwah, NJ: Lawrence Erlbaum.

Ashforth, B.E., & Mael, F. (1989). Social identity theory and the organization. *Academy of Management Review, 14,* 20–39.

Ashmore, R. D., Deaux, K., & McLaughlin-Volpe, T. (2004). An organizing framework for collective identity: Articulation and significance of multidimensionality. *Psychological Bulletin, 130,* 80–114.

Bagger, J., Li, A., & Gutek, B.A. (2008). How much do you value your family and does it matter? The joint effects of family identity salience, family-interference-with-work, and gender. *Human Relations, 61,* 187–211.

Beehr, T.A., & Glazer, S. (2001). A cultural perspective of social support in relation to occupational stress. In P.L. Perrewé & D.C. Ganster (Eds.), *Research in occupational stress and well being* (Vol. 1, pp. 97–102). Oxford, UK: Elsevier Science.

Brown, M.E. (1969). Identification and some conditions of organizational involvement. *Administrative Science Quarterly, 14,* 346–355.

Callero, P.L. (1985). Role-identity salience. *Social Psychology Quarterly, 48,* 203–214.

Clark, R. A., Nye, F. I., & Gecas, V. (1978). Husbands' work involvement and marital role performance. *Journal of Marriage and the Family, 40,* 9–21.

Cohen, S., & Wills, T.A. (1985). Stress, social support, and buffering hypothesis, *Psychological Review, 98,* 310–357.

Das, D., Dharwadkar, R., & Brandes, P. (2008). The importance of being 'Indian': Identity centrality and work outcomes in an off-shored call center in India. *Human Relations, 61,* 1499–1530.

Deaux, K. (1996). Social identification. In E.T. Higgins & A.W. Kruglanski (Eds.), *Social psychology: Handbook of basic principles* (pp. 777–798). New York, NY: Guilford Press.

Dutton, J.E., Dukerich, J.M., & Harquail, C. V. (1994). Organizational images and member identification. *Administrative Science Quarterly, 39,* 239–263.

Foddy, M., & Kashima, Y. (2002). Self and identity: What is the conception of the person assumed in the current literature? In Y. Kashima, M. Foddy, & M. Platow (Eds.), *Self and identity: Personal, social, and symbolic* (pp. 3–25). Mahwah, NJ: Lawrence Erlbaum Associates.

Folkman, S., & Lazarus, R.S. (1985). If it changes it must be a process: Study of emotion and coping during three stages of a college examination. *Journal of Personality and Social Psychology, 48,* 150–170.

Folkman, S., & Lazarus, R.S. (1988). Coping as a mediator of emotion. *Journal of Personality and Social Psychology, 54,* 466–475.

Ganster, D.C., Fusilier, M.R., & Mayes, B.T. (1986). Role of social support in the experience of stress at work. *Journal of Applied Psychology, 71,* 102–110.

Hogg, M.A., & Terry, D.J. (2001). *Social identity process in organizational contexts.* Philadelphia, PA: Psychology Press.

Kanter, R.M. (1977). Some effects of proportions on group life: Skewed sex ratios and responses to token women. *American Journal of Sociology, 82*, 965–990.

Kreiner, G.E., Hollensbe, E.C., & Sheep, M.L. (2006). Where is the "me" among the "we"? Identity work and the search for optimal balance. *Academy of Management Journal, 49*, 1031–1057.

Kreiner, G.E., & Ashforth, B.E. (2004). Evidence toward an expanded model of organizational identification. *Journal of Organizational Behavior, 25*, 1–27.

Lazarus, R.S. (1993). From psychological stress to the emotions: A history of changing outlooks. *Annual Review of Psychology, 44*, 1–21.

Lazarus, R.S., & Folkman, S. (1987). Transactional theory and research on emotions and coping. *European Journal of Personality, 1*, 141–169.

Lewin, K. (1936). *A dynamic theory of personality.* New York, NY: McGraw-Hill.

Markus, H. (1977). Self—Schemata and processing information about the self. *Journal of Personality and Social Psychology, 35*, 63–78.

McCall, G. J., & Simmons, J. L. (1978). *Identities and interactions* (rev. ed.). New York, NY: Free Press.

Mead, G. H. (1934). *Mind, self, and society.* Chicago, IL: University of Chicago Press.

Mehra, A., Kilduff, M., & Brass, D.J. (1998). At the margins: A distinctiveness approach to the social identity and social networks of underrepresented groups. *Academy of Management Journal, 41*, 441–452.

Merton, R. K. (1957). *Social theory and social structure* (rev. ed.). New York, NY: Free Press.

Meurs, J.A. & Perrewé, P.L. (2011). Cognitive activation theory of stress: An integrative theoretical approach to work stress. *Journal of Management, 37*, 1043–1066.

Perrewé, P.L., & Zellars, K.L. (1999). An examination of attributions and emotions in the transactional approach to the organizational stress process. *Journal of Organizational Behavior, 20*, 739–752.

Segal, L.M., & Sullivan, D.G. (1997). The growth of temporary services work. *Journal of Economic Perspectives, 11*, 117–136.

Stryker, S. (1980). *Symbolic interactionism: A social structural version.* Menlo Park, CA: Benjamin/Cummings.

Stryker, S., & Burke, P. J. (2000). The past, present, and future of an identity theory. *Social Psychology Quarterly, 63*, 284–297.

Stryker, S., & Serpe, R.T. (1982). Commitment, identity salience, and role behavior: A theory and research example. In W. Ickes & E.S. Knowles (Eds.), *Personality, roles, and social behavior* (pp. 199–218). New York, NY: Springer-Verlag.

Stryker, S., & Serpe, R.T. (1994). Identity salience and psychological centrality: Equivalent, overlapping, or complementary concepts? *Social Psychology Quarterly, 57*, 16–35.

Tajfel, H. (1972). La catégoristion sociale (Social categorization). In S. Moscovici (Ed.), *Introduction á la psychologie sociale* (Vol. 1, pp. 272–302). Paris, France: Larousse.

van Knippenberg, D. (2000). Work motivation and performance: A social identity perspective. *Applied Psychology: An Interactional Review, 49*, 357–371.

Verbrugge, L. M. (1983). Multiple roles and physical health of women and mean. *Journal of Health and Social Behavior, 24*, 16–30.

Viswesvaran, C., Sanchez, J.I., & Fisher, J. (1999). The role of social support in the process of work stress: A meta-analysis. *Journal of Vocational Behavior, 54*, 314–334.

Washington, S.K. (2000). *The role-based identity scale: Development and field tests involving stock options and skill-based pay applications.* Doctoral dissertation, Cornell University, Ithaca, NY.

CHAPTER 3

THE RELATIONSHIP BETWEEN STRESS, ALCOHOL USE, AND WORK

Edilaine C. Silva Gherardi-Donato, Margarita Antonia Villar Luis, and Clarissa Mendonça Corradi-Webster

The term *stress* can be defined as a process that involves the perception, integration, response, and adaptation to aversive, threatening, or challenging events. It is a philogenetically old stereotyped adaptation pattern designed to prepare the body for physical activity (Seyle, 1975).

In the body subjected to strong strain, a long biochemical process is triggered as a result of the activation of the hypothalamic-pituitary-adrenal axis (HPA) and the sympathetic nervous system. Firstly, there is a hormonal mobilization designed to strengthen the body and as a result of the activation of the sympathetic nervous system, there is an increase in heart rate, blood glucose levels, pupil dilation, and respiratory stimulation. These physiological changes occur, as has already been mentioned, to prepare the body to fight or flee from the stressor and maintain homeostasis.

This emergency response process has been following humans in their evolutionary history, and the theory advanced by Selye proposes three

Coping and Prevention, pages 43–52

changes in the body that explain the symptoms that occur in the stress response. These changes were discovered from his laboratory research and later extrapolated, with some adaptations, to the human body. In 1956, Selye established that stress is developed in three phases: alarm, resistance, and exhaustion. When reviewing these concepts in 1984, Selye suggested that the body always tried to adapt to stressful events using, in the process, large amounts of adaptive energy.

According to this theory, in the alarm phase, the body is prepared for the life-saving fight-or-flight response. If stress remains for an undetermined period of time, the resistance phase starts, when the body tries to adapt (in its tendency to maintain internal homeostasis) and then a feeling of wear and tiredness emerges. If the stressor continues to affect a body that lacks strategies to cope with the stress that is generated, it depletes the reserves of adaptive energy, triggering the exhaustion phase, a period during which severe illnesses can emerge.

We know that stressful situations can evoke a number of responses that can be broken down into two types: stress itself and coping. According to Lazarus and Folkman (1984), responses that emerge spontaneously belong to the former type; these are involuntary responses triggered by stressful stimuli. Those responses that are evoked by the same stimuli but which remain due to their consequences are characteristic of coping. These consequences are related both to changes in the external environment and to the effects on aversive conditions in the body itself.

For these authors, coping is processed through the mobilization of natural resources aiming at dealing with stressful situations and it consists of the interaction between the body and the environment, in which a set of strategies is used to promote adaptation to stressful circumstances. Cognitive and behavioral efforts come into play to cope with demands that exceed the resources the individual currently has.

In an effort to cope with stressful situations, individuals use coping strategies, which Lazarus and Folkman (1984) have defined as belonging to two types: problem-focused coping and emotion-focused coping. The first type of strategy is addressed to changing situations and the latter to unchangeable situations; coping strategies are deliberate, organic or not, and occurring as a response to an identified stressor.

Therefore, in the view of these authors, coping has two functions: changing the relationship between individuals and the environment, by controlling or changing the problem that is causing the discomfort (problem-focused coping), and adapting the emotional response to the problem (emotion-focused coping). The forms of emotion-focused coping occur more frequently when individuals think that nothing can be done to change a damaging situation, environmental threat, or challenge. On the other hand, the forms of problem-focused coping are more likely to occur when conditions are considered amenable to change. Both forms of coping mutually influence each other as individuals deal with stressful situations, which may preclude or facilitate the emergence of either of them.

The perception individuals have that they can control the situation partially determines how they assess situations as amenable to change through actions taken by them. This assessment has an impact on the coping responses individuals will resort to, because if they feel unable to act upon a given stressor, they will probably use strategies that are more compatible with their inability and, therefore, included in the emotion-focused coping category. On the other hand, individuals who think they can have a reasonable control over situations will prefer problem-focused coping (Hunziker, 1997).

STRESS AND THE USE OF PSYCHOACTIVE SUBSTANCES AND THE RELATIONSHIP WITH WORK

Studies conducted in the 1990s (Cooper, Russel, Skinner, & Frone, 1992; Corcoran & Stern, 1994) found that alcohol use was a successful coping response used in avoidance to mitigate, ward off, or end aversive situations in the public or private sphere. When coping with stress, some individuals who are subject to an overload of stressors or who are about to be exposed to aversive situations may resort to drinking as a way to try to reduce their strain levels. Alcohol use to regulate emotions under stressful situations is an example of emotion-focused coping strategies.

In the past few years, stress has been identified as a significant factor leading people to start and continue to use psychoactive substances, among them alcohol, in addition to playing a role in substance use relapse (Goeders, 2003; Weiss, 2005).

The abusive use of alcohol is not just a consequence of organic causes, but rather of a set of biological, psychological, and social factors. Therefore, the role played by work in the development of the abusive use of this substance should be considered, and we should also analyze the relationship between occupational stress and the consumption of psychoactive substances.

In Brazil, alcoholism is the third most frequent reason for work absenteeism, the most frequent cause of early retirement and occupational accidents, and the eighth most frequent cause of sick pay paid by the Social Security Department (Vaissman, 2004). Additionally, it may cause delays, decreased productivity, material waste, sleepiness, conflicts with coworkers, conflicts with supervisors, difficulties understanding new instructions and recognizing mistakes, overreaction to criticism, and mood swings (Vaissman, 2004).

Stress is a common human experience and one that is needed, driving people to meet their basic needs, perform daily activities, and go for their dreams and desires. However, certain settings may cause high levels of stress, making individuals suffer—one of them being the workplace.

Considering the way modern society and work relations are organized today, there are many situations that may be conducive to stress. Among these situations are the effects and consequences of the increasing urbanization process, long work days or shift work, worsening in labor relations, the demands of flexible specialization (production reengineering) with workers having to constantly change, demands for greater production, and competitiveness at work, among others (Sennett, 1998).

One of the models used to assess stress in the workplace was proposed in the 1970s by Robert Karasek (Karasek & Theorell, 1990), which is known as the Demand-Control Model. According to this model, stress in the workplace is a result of the interaction between high physical and psychological demands, less control in the work production process and in decision-making, and less social support from coworkers and supervisors (Alves, 2004).

People who are more vulnerable to strain would have a small repertoire of social and personal resources to adaptively respond to stressful situations at work. Added to that is the fact that they have positive expectations regarding the effects of alcohol, having been through situations in which they felt more relaxed after drinking, thus avoiding the negative emotion of stress. Therefore, they include alcohol consumption in their repertoire of stress-coping strategies, using it repeatedly in future situations. Literature also shows that people learn how to drink to manage stress by observing the behavior of people close to them. Individuals whose parents drink heavily and who use alcohol to reduce stress at work also seem to adopt such a behavior in order to cope with adverse situations (Moore, Sikora, Grunberg, & Greenberg, 2007).

Some studies have used the above-mentioned model and have found a relationship with the use of psychoactive substances. People who work in environments with high (physical or psychological) demand and little control over the production process will be at a higher risk of becoming drug addicts (Reed, Storr, & Anthony, 2006). A high psychological demand seems to play a key role in occupational stress. Crum, Muntaner, Eaton, and Anthony (1995) found that men who are subject to high psychological demand and who had little control over their work were 27.5 times more likely to develop the behavior of alcohol abuse or dependence. Regarding high physical demand and little control over work, these authors found that the likelihood of developing alcohol use-related disorders increased 3.4 times.

Among the factors that may cause an overload at work and increase the likelihood of drinking are the following: stress, work organization, interpersonal relationship issues, availability of the substances at the workplace or in its surroundings, and long time away from the family (Niel, 2008). Although there is a scarcity of studies in the field of occupational stress and drug use, stress has emerged as a potential risk factor for alcohol abuse or dependence (Frone, 2008). Therefore, the workplace becomes an important target for prevention activities. Considering the statistics and the costs resulting from days away from work, delays and disability retirement, in addition to workers' health problems and how this all can affect their quality of life, further studies on the relationship between work and alcohol use and stress are warranted.

In the framework of prevention at the workplace, the authors decided to investigate the relationship between alcohol use and occupational stress. Since 2003 the authors, with the help of a professional who specializes in chemical dependence, had been carrying out a counseling activity with workers in general and a support activity for chemically dependent workers from sectors connected to the central administration of a public university located in the city of Ribeirão Preto, State of São Paulo.

The first step of this study at this location was conducted in 2008, at the Central Campus Administration, which has 390 workers working in several areas (administration, technical maintenance, parks and gardens, healthcare). Workers were formally invited to participate in the study, and they were given the required explanations about the research. The study sample consists of 149 individuals who accepted to participate. The data collection instruments included the Social-Demographic Data Questionnaire (QSD), the Standard Questionnaire on the Pattern of Alcohol Use (AUDIT), and the Job Stress Scale. The Social-Demographic Data Questionnaire included questions related to the individual's identification, economic status, education, religion, and information on the role performed in the job.

The questionnaire used to screen for health conditions related to alcohol use, the AUDIT, was developed by the World Health Organization (Babor, Fuente, Saunders, & Grant, 1992) and translated and validated in Brazil (Lima, Freire, Silva, Teixeira, Farrell, & Prince, 2005). The purpose of this instrument is to identify individuals with patterns of hazardous drinking, harmful alcohol use and alcohol dependence. AUDIT consists of 10 questions that assess alcohol consumption in the past 12 months. The first three items measure the amount and frequency of regular alcohol use. The next three questions check for dependence symptoms and the four last questions are related to recent life issues that could be related to alcohol consumption. The scale ranges from 0 to 40, showing the individual's drinking pattern. According to the literature, this instrument is very useful in screening for hazardous drinking and alcohol-related problems because it is standardized and has been translated and validated in Brazil; it is short, easy to use, and flexible, providing information that will be used to give feedback to respondents; it is in accordance with CID-10 regarding harmful drinking and dependence and is focused on recent alcohol use (Babor & Higgle-Biddle, 2003).

The Job Stress Scale—JSS—is made up of items that assess the demand, control and social support related to stress at the workplace. The interpretation of the scores is specific for each of the scale items, with increasing stress levels and the scores increase on the scale which, in turn, indicates greater Demand, less Control and greater Social Support. The scale has been translated and validated for use in Brazil (Alves, Chor, Faerstein, & Lopes, 2004).

As for participants' demographics, 74.3% were females, 59.2% lived with their family, 63.8% were married or lived with their partner, 64.5% had children who lived with them, 52.6% had a college degree, 62.5% were Catholic, and 48.7% had jobs that required a high school degree. The average age of the sample was 44.3 years (SD = 8.54; min = 23, max = 61). Average family income was R$4,238 (SD = 2,231; min = 800, max = 12,000).

The results of the Job Stress Scale showed an average of 12.8 for the Demand item (SD = 3.68; min = 0, max = 19), an average of 17.7 for the Control item (SD = 4.09; min = 0, max = 24), and an average of 19.8 for the Social Support item (SD = 4.78; min = 0, max = 24).

The first question asked in the AUDIT, on the frequency of alcohol consumption, showed that 32.9% drink once a month or less. The second question is related to the number of drinks people usually have when they drink, showing that 53.8% had one drink. Regarding how often they had five drinks or more on one occasion, asked in question number three, 32.9% answered they would drink as much in one occasion. The fourth question is related to the number of occasions in the past year when they found that they could not stop drinking once they had started, 4.9% responded positively. The fifth question asked how often in the past year individuals had failed to do what was expected of them because of drinking, 3.5% answered positively. When asked, in question number six, how often during the past year they had needed a drink in the morning to get themselves going after a heavy drinking session the previous day, 100% of the subjects answer never. Regarding feeling guilt or remorse, also during the past year, after drinking (question number seven), 9.9% answered positively. Question number eight asked if during the past year individuals had been unable to remember what had happened the night before because they had been drinking, 6.3% answered positively. When asked, in question number nine, if they or someone else had been injured as a result of their drinking, 3.5% answered positively. And, finally, in question number ten, they were asked if a relative, friend, or doctor had been concerned about their drinking or suggested they cut down, with 6.3% giving positive answers.

The scoring in the AUDIT was classified according to cutoff points to establish the consumption pattern, and we found that most individuals had a score that classifies them as low-risk alcohol consumers (89.5%). However, 9.1% of individuals fit in the hazardous drinking category, a fact that highlights the importance of educational actions at the workplace and the implementation of measures to reduce the risk. Regarding harmful drinking and possible dependence, we found that 0.7% of individuals exhibited both patterns, thus reinforcing the fact that the previously mentioned intervention measures should be adopted. The average AUDIT score was 3.15 (SD = 3.7; min = 0; max = 23).

Additional questions on alcohol use were included in the instrument in order to get complementary information that enabled us to investigate drinking-related problems. In the sample, only 5.3% stated they had ever had drinking-related problems; among those quoted by the respondents, 62.5% were physical (headache, dizziness, memory loss, and weight gain), and 37.5% were psychosocial (spouse felt bothered and interference in personal relationships, forgetting what they had done after drinking). In spite of the problems mentioned, none of the individuals reported they had ever looked for help to solve their drinking issues. As for getting information on alcohol consumption, 19.7% of the subjects said they would be interested in it, thus reinforcing the importance of educational programs at the workplace.

In the sample of campus workers, we found a relationship between alcohol use and the control individuals had at their work environment, so that the less control individuals had, and therefore the greater the stress they experienced, the higher the score in the alcohol use questionnaire (Spearman; $r = 0.28$; $p < 0.001$). However, this relationship was not found in the demand and social support items, which shows the need to conduct studies targeted at the control dimension or at the combination of these job stress dimensions.

OUTLOOK FOR PREVENTION AND TREATMENT

Prevention in the workplace is considered important, since this is the place where individuals spend most of their day, in addition to being an environment that can contribute to increasing stress levels. Although the most serious triggering factors are usually found outside the work environment, most people who have hazardous or harmful drinking behavior work, thus spending most of their time at work. Therefore, the workplace is a favorable place to implement actions designed to decrease the incidence and reduce the consumption of substances, in addition to being an important place from which to refer individuals to specialized services and should also provide them support at times of relapse (Crum, Muntaner, Eaton, & Anthony, 1995).

Considering that work relationships and processes can cause stress and that this stress can increase the chances of alcohol consumption, services designed to prevent the consumption of this substance should approach the factors that cause stress. One suggestion is not to approach the issue of alcohol use as an isolated problem, but rather deal with it at a more holistic level, gearing actions towards workers' health (Griep, Chor, & Camacho, 1998).

In this framework, researchers with the Nursing School of Ribeirão Preto at the São Paulo University linked to the Department of Psychiatric Nursing and Human Sciences have been working on research projects on the relationship between job stress and the use of psychoactive substances. The research proposal involves graduate and undergraduate students, employees, and professors. The problematic use of alcohol among workers was the starting point for the activities by the research group who found that one single approach was not enough to meet workers' demands, therefore showing in practice that this issue should be approached within a specific context and from different dimensions.

Today, efforts are being made to map this problem throughout the university campus, and the above-mentioned research project in addition to screening the use of legal substances could also strengthen the links with all workers by getting to know the characteristics of their workplaces and including their diversity in terms of role, education, purchasing power, and exposure to psychological demands that can generate stress.

The research work as well as the experience provided by the workers' counseling and support program have generated sound knowledge that can be used as a foundation for future projects that include the use of alternative strategies designed to expand the repertoire of healthy behaviors to manage stress, be it at the workplace or in other social contexts of these workers and, as a result, improve their quality of life. Considering research results that found that stress is an important factor that leads people to start and continue the use of psychoactive substances and one that can trigger relapse in users undergoing treatment and adding this knowledge to the literature that demonstrates that the work setting is an increasingly demanding and hostile environment for people, this study shows the need for greater investments in research on the relationship between stress, alcohol use, and work.

ACKNOWLEDGEMENT

Research project funded by FAPESP (Research Funding Agency of the State of São Paulo) Process: 2009/00457-5.

REFERENCES

Alves, M.G.M., Chor, D., Faerstein, E., & Lopes, C.S. (2004). Short version of the "job stress scale": A Portuguese-language adaptation. *Revista de Saúde Pública, 38,* 164–172.

Babor, T.F., Fuente, J.R., Saunders, J., & Grant, M. (1992). AUDIT: The alcohol use disorders identification test: guidelines for use in primary health care. *WHO (World Health Organization)/PAHO, 4,* 1–29.

Babor, T. F., & Higgle-Biddle, J. C. (2003). *Intervenções breves para uso de risco e nocivo de álcool: manual para uso em atenção primária – Tradução CM Corradi.* Ribeirão Preto, Brasil: PAI-PAD, SP.

Cooper, M.L., Russel, M., Skinner, J.B., & Frone, M.R. (1992). Stress and alcohol use: Moderating effects of gender coping and alcohol expectancies. *Journal of Abnormal Psychology. 101*(1), 139–152.

Corcoran, G.D., & Stern, M. (1994). Predicting reduction in tension following alcohol consumption in a stressful situation with the alcohol expectancy questionnaire. *Addictive Behaviour, 19*(1), 57–62.

Crum, R. M., Muntaner, C., Eaton, W. W., & Anthony, J. C. (1995). Occupational stress and the risk of alcohol-abuse and dependence. *Alcoholism-Clinical and Experimental Research, 19*(3), 647–655.

Frone, M.R., (2008). Are work stressors related to employee substance use? The importance of temporal context assessments of alcohol and illicit drug use. *Journal of Applied Psychology, 93(*1), 199–206.

Goeders, N.E. (2003). The impacto f stress on addiction. *Eur Neuropsychofarmacology,* Amsterdam, *13,* 435–441.

Griep, R. H., Chor, D., & Camacho, L. B. (1998). Tabagismo entre trabalhadores de empresa bancária. *Revista de Saúde Pública. 32*(6), 533–540.

Hunziker, M.H.L. (1997).Um olhar crítico sobre o estudo do desamparo aprendido. *Estudo de psicologia, 14*(3), 17–26.

Karasek, R. & Theorell, T. (1990). *Healthy work: Stress, productivity and the reconstruction of working life.* New York, NY: Basic Books.

Lazarus, R.S., & Folkman, S. (1984). *Stress, appraisal, & coping.* New York, NY: Springer.

Lima, C. Freire, A.C.C., Silva, A.P.B., Teixeira, R.M., Farrell, M., & Prince, M. (2005). Concurrent and construct validity of the audit in an urban Brazilian sample. *Alcohol, 40,* 584–589.

Moore, S., Sikora, P., Grunberg, L., & Greenberg, E. (2007). Work stress and alcohol use: Examining the tension-reduction model as a function of worker's parent's alcohol use. *Addictive Behavior, 32*(12), 3114–3121.

Niel, M. (2008). Alcoolismo no trabalho. Programa de Orientação e Atendimentos a Dependentes – PROAD. Retrieved from http://ww2.prefeitura.sp.gov.br//arquivos/secretarias/gestaopublica/servidores/desat/0012/alcool_empresa.pdf

Reed, P. L., Storr, C. L., & Anthony, J. C. (2006). Drug dependence environments: Job strain in the work environment and risk of becoming drug-dependent. *American Journal of Epidemiology, 163*(5), 404–411.

Sennett, R. (1998). *The corrosion of character: The personal consequences of work in the new capitalism.* New York, NY: W. W. Norton & Company.

Selye, H. (1975). Confusion and controversy in the stress field. *Journal of Human Stress, 1,* 37–44.

Selye, H. (1984). History and present status of the stress concept. In S. Breznitz & L. Goldberger (Eds), *Handbook of stress: Theoretical and clinical aspects* (pp. 7–20). New York, NY: The Free Press.

Vaissman, M. (2004). *Alcoolismo no trabalho.* Rio de Janeiro, Brasil: Editora Garamond.

Weiss, F. (2005). Neurobiology of craving, conditioned reward and relapse. *Current Opnion Pharmacology, 5,* 9–19.

CHAPTER 4

AGE-RELATED TRENDS IN WORKERS' SUBJECTIVE WELL-BEING AND PERCEIVED JOB QUALITY[1]

Jessica M. Streit
National Institute for Occupational Safety & Health

Steven L. Sauter
Consultant to the Office of the Director, National Institute for Occupational Safety & Health

Dennis J. Hanseman
Department of Environmental Health University of Cincinnati

The aging of the labor force is a well-documented phenomenon in developed countries around the world. In the U.S., this trend is associated with two events: (1) the aging of the baby boomer cohort, and (2) the early 1990s reversal of the long-term decline in labor force participation rates for individuals over 55 (Mosisa & Hipple, 2006). In the period 2005–2020, the number of U.S. workers aged 55 years and older is expected to increase

Coping and Prevention, pages 53–71

from just over 24 million to nearly 40 million. This represents an average annual growth rate of 4.2%, compared to virtually no growth (0.20%) for workers in the younger 25–54 year age group or the workforce overall (0.76%; Toosi, 2006).

Developed countries experiencing this type of worker demographic shift, including the U.S., have created new priorities in response to it. Especially in countries with little overall population growth, further attention will need to be given to ways to retain their older workforce members to sustain national economies. Additionally, there is a growing need to give greater attention to designing jobs that older persons can continue to safely and effectively perform. This is both a social imperative and a precondition for retaining older workers.

Efforts to control levels of job stress faced by older workers may be an important measure for addressing these priorities. A large body of research documents age-related declines in physical and psychological functioning, including decrements in strength and endurance; sensory and psychomotor function; and aspects of cognitive functioning like cognitive speed, memory, and novel problem solving (Wegman & McGee, 2004). These declines raise the possibility that demanding conditions in today's workplace—including long work hours, lean production technologies, and rapid technological change—may be especially stressful for older workers and even place them at higher risk for illness and injury (Barnes-Farrell, 2005; Griffiths, 2007; Kowalski-Trakofler, Steiner, & Schwerha, 2005; NRC, 2004). However, research addressing age differentials in sensitivity to workplace exposures is sparse, and one popular conjecture is that risks associated with declining function might be offset by older workers' accumulated skills and experiences, compensatory strategies, and improved coping styles (Barnes-Farrell, 2005; Griffiths, 2007, Kowalski-Trakofler et al., 2005; Robertson & Tracy, 1998; Wegman & McGee, 2004). A review of literature conducted by the National Research Council (NRC; Wegman & McGee, 2004) cites this offset hypothesis and found that, at least for performance outcomes, acquired experience may not fully compensate for effects of age-related declines.

In addition to the risks stress may pose to the health and safety of older workers, accumulating literature also points to an influence of stressful working conditions on older persons' early withdrawal from the workforce. Pioneering studies on "workability" by the Finnish National Institute of Occupational Health have looked broadly at workplace factors contributing to aging workers' declining capacities and ensuing disability retirements. Of interest, these studies found that conditions commonly recognized as risk or protective factors for job stress (esteem, recognition, and supervisory relationships) were strong predictors of work capacity (Tuomi et al., 1997; Tuomi, Ilmarinen, Martikainen, Aalto, & Klockars, 1997).

Results from other investigations in Scandinavia and Europe complement these findings. In a Finnish study of workers in the health and social services sector, high levels of job demands and low levels of job control were both separately and interactively predictive of early retirement thoughts (Elovainio, Forma, Kivimäki, Sinervo, Sutinen, & Laine, 2005). Similarly, an analysis of data from nearly 7,000 participants in the first round of the European Survey of Health, Aging and Retirement also found that that stressful working conditions (defined by low control and effort–reward imbalance) predicted early retirement intentions (Siegrist, Wahrendorf, von dem Knesebeck, Jürges, & Börsch-Supan, 2006). Other European work has linked stressful conditions with actual retirement, not just intentions to retire. Organizational restructuring and routine, unchallenging tasks were both associated with early retirement in a 1994 study of civil servants in the Netherlands (Hennekens & Tazelaar, 1994). Job dissatisfaction was predictive of retirement in the prospective study of British civil servants enrolled in the Whitehall II study (Mein, Martikainen, Stansfeld, Brunner, Fuhrer, & Marmot, 2000).

Assuming that stressful working conditions do pose a risk to the health and safety of older workers (whether or not the risks are elevated in comparison to younger workers' risks) and that such conditions lead to early withdrawal from the workforce, the question of interest becomes: *how stressful is the work situation for older workers?* Evidence from credible sources like the General Social Survey (GSS) suggest that today's workplaces, in general, are surprisingly stressful. Data from recent waves of the GSS reveal that nearly one third of all workers view their jobs as "often" or "always" stressful, though older workers do report somewhat lower frequencies of job stress than younger workers do (Davis, Smith, & Marsden, 2002).

The purpose of this chapter is to broadly examine the evidence on risks of job stress among older workers and better gauge risks to their health and workforce retention. An exhaustive review of the relevant literature is beyond the scope and intention of this chapter; rather, we try to provide a representative sampling of pertinent research, including studies of pivotal significance and a summary of recent National Institute for Occupational Safety and Health (NIOSH) investigations on this topic. We begin with an overview of research on comparative levels of reported job stress and other aspects of subjective well-being among workers of different ages as an indirect measure of stressful working conditions among older workers. We then turn to a smaller body of research on age differences in reported exposures to job quality factors that are associated with job stress as a more direct indicator of stressful working conditions among older workers.

AGE DIFFERENCES IN THE SUBJECTIVE WELL-BEING OF OLDER WORKERS

Age and reported levels of job stress are our primary focus, but mental health outcomes (mainly anxiety and depression) and job satisfaction are worth mentioning in order to broadly characterize workers' age-related affective changes potentially influenced by the quality of work. Research on this topic encompasses a range of occupation-specific studies and broader representative surveys employing both simple descriptive analyses and multivariable statistical strategies and also sometimes exploring possible higher-order age effects. Our review of this work begins with narrower studies and proceeds to the more complex investigations. Overall, it shows a rather positive picture emerging for older workers: The bulk of the evidence provides little or no indication that subjective well-being deteriorates with age. On the contrary, the studies more commonly suggest that older workers experience reduced levels of job stress and improved overall mental health and job satisfaction levels in comparison to younger workers.

Job Stress

Findings from both occupation-specific investigations and findings from large representative surveys suggest that job stress levels decline for older workers. However, these results are a bit uneven, and stronger evidence of this trend comes from studies in the U.S. than from European research. An occupation-specific study of work experiences of middle-aged (30–53 years) and preretirement-aged (54–72 years) white-collar workers in the U.S. by Remondet and Hansson (1991), for example, found that older workers report significantly less job tension/stress and reduced generalized stress than younger workers. Similarly, age-related reductions in reported stress are reported in an occupation-specific study of Scottish physicians (Swanson, Power, & Simpson, 1996).

Recent NIOSH analyses of data from more representative worker surveys further support these findings. We observed a trend toward reduced stress among older workers in analyses of data from the 2004 wave of the Health and Retirement Survey (HRS) conducted by the University of Michigan. The HRS is a biennial survey of 22,000 workers aged 50 and older (Sauter, Streit, & Hanseman, 2009). Agreement with the survey item "my job involves a lot of stress" declines across age strata in the sample, from 63% for workers aged 51–64 years, to 39% for workers aged 65–74 years, to 27% for workers older than 74. We also found a similar age gradient in reported job stress in analyses of data from the 2002 NIOSH Quality of Work Life Survey (QWL) (Sauter et al., 2009). The QWL is administered as a module of the

GSS and captures data on occupational health and job quality from nearly 1,800 working U.S. adults. Unlike the descriptive analyses dominating studies of age and stress, we employed hierarchical regression techniques in our analyses of the QWL data, controlling for a variety of demographic factors (gender, education, race, marital status) and job attributes (tenure, status, self-employment, home work, full- or part-time work, multiple job holding) when investigating associations of age with stress and other outcomes. Even after controlling for these, we still found a significant monotonic decline in the frequency ("always" to "never") with which workers aged 18–89 years reported work as stressful.

In contrast to the trend toward declining stress among older workers seen in both occupation-specific studies and the broader NIOSH investigations, the results of several large European surveys provide a more complex picture of the age-stress trend. Smith (2001), for example, observed an association between age and stress in over 4,000 workers sampled from the Bristol (UK) electoral register. In this case, the relationship appears to be curvilinear, not monotonic, in nature. Workers aged 41–50 years in this sample were the most likely (21%) to report feeling "very" or "extremely" stressed at work. In comparison, just 17% of workers 50 years or older reported such high levels of stress—a rate very close to the rate for high levels of stress for workers aged 18–32 years (16%). Also, in a recent expansive review of the literature on the health of aging workers, Griffiths, Knight, and Mohd Mahudin (2009) reported that a frequent finding in age and job stress research is that workers in their 40s and 50s are the age group to report the highest job-related stress levels.

Data from the British Labour Force Surveys further highlight these age–stress complexities and also bring to light the complications with defining "older workers." The British Labour Force Survey is a quarterly survey of 60,000 UK households and is the primary vehicle in the UK for gathering data on work-related illness and injury in the British workforce. Griffiths (2007) reported results from the 2004–2005 survey showing that stress, depression, and anxiety are among the most populated categories of work-related illness, and these conditions are more prevalent among older (aged 45 years to retirement) than younger workers (under 45 years). Conversely, when the Labour Force Surveys of 2004–2005 to 2007–2008 were assessed collectively, Griffiths et al. (2009) discovered a relatively flat, inverse u-shaped relationship between age and the three work-related illnesses. Here, workers aged 35–54 years had the highest self-reported levels of stress, depression, and anxiety, and workers aged 55 years and older had the lowest levels (with workers 34 years and younger in between). Further exploration of this relationship, however, discovered little difference between workers 34–60 years old but found a decrease in anxiety, depression, and stress in workers over 60.

Finally, no age–stress trend is found at all in data from the Third European Survey of Working Conditions, which captures data from nearly 16,000 workers from EU15 countries. Ilmarinen (2005) reported that analyses of health data from this survey fail to show EU15-wide differences in the prevalence of work-related "psychosomatic syndrome" (affirmative response to one or more items pertaining to stress and tension, general fatigue, sleeping disorders, anxiety, irritability, or mental trauma) between workers under and over 45 years of age. There are also no age differences in the prevalence of "stress syndrome" (affirmative response to one or more items denoting head- and stomachache, stress, general fatigue, or tension). However, it is worth considering whether or not the age split chosen for these analyses might be masking notable trends. To illustrate this possibility, it is plausible that age effects may also have been absent in the Smith (2001) study had the sample been split at age 45 because of the symmetrical downturn in stress for individuals both younger and older than 41–50 years.

Mental Health

In comparison to studies of age and stress outcomes, there is stronger concurrence among studies of age and mental health outcomes that increasing age is protective of subjective well-being among workers. The outcomes investigated in many of these studies are context-free measures of mental health, however. Therefore, attribution to the workplace may be less certain than for job stress and job satisfaction outcomes.

A study of 634 Hong Kong managers aged 20–72 years by Siu, Spector, Cooper, and Donald (2001), for instance, found that older workers exhibit improved mental well-being as it is measured on the Occupational Stress Indicator-2 (Williams & Cooper, 1996). Declines in depression and anxiety among older workers also appear in several additional studies. The older cohort (aged 54–72 years) in Remondet and Hansson's (1991) study of white collar workers had significantly lower scores on the Center for Epidemiologic Studies Depression Scale (CES-D) than did the younger cohort (aged 30–53 years). Similarly, Frone, Russell, and Barnes (1996) reported significant negative correlations between age and CES-D scores among employed parents in two studies of work-family conflict using data from large random community samples.

Analyses of data from representative surveys of workers support the age trends in mental health seen in these narrower studies. Most recently, a study of more than 60,000 workers from large private and public organizations in Australia uncovered age-related declines in self-reported psychological distress as measured by the Kessler-6 component of the World Health Organization's Health and Performance at Work Questionnaire (Hilton et al., 2008).

Additionally, data from the Canadian Community Health Survey were used to examine the age distribution in major depressive episodes from a weighted sample of nearly 750,000 Canadian workers (Blackmore et al., 2007). Analyses of these data showed the odds of depression for workers significantly declining across age strata, from 18–24 years to 35–44 years to 55+ years.

Our own analyses of HRS and QWL data also show age-related declines in mental health problems among workers (Sauter et al., 2009). Analyses of the 2004 HRS revealed a lower 12-month prevalence of two or more weeks of feeling sad, blue, or depressed among workers aged 65–74 years (7%) than those aged 51–64 years (22%). Unlike the continuing decline seen in reported stress among the oldest HRS cohort, however, the prevalence rate for these dysphoric states increases among workers older than 74 (17%). Additional examination of the age pattern in mental health using a question taken from the Centers for Disease Control and Prevention (CDC) Behavioral Risk Factor Surveillance Survey, which asked survey participants to report the number of days in the last 30 days their mental health (including stress, depression, and problems with emotions) was not good (CDC, 2000). Similar to the monotonic age trend we saw for the QWL job stress measure, we found a significant, age-related, linear decline for this mental health indicator.

Finally, similar to the curvilinear age–stress relationship reported by Smith (2001), analyses of data from two large British surveys found curvilinear relationships between age and mental health indicators. In a study of nearly 1,700 employed British adults, Warr (1992) found workers in early middle age have higher levels of anxiety and depression than either younger or older workers. Although these two curvilinear effects became nonsignificant when other possible explanatory or mediating variables were added to Warr's analyses, significant linear relationships remained, depicting decreases in depression and anxiety as age increased. Analysis of General Health Questionnaire scores from over 5,000 employed participants in the 1991 British Household Panel Study also revealed a curvilinear effect of age on mental health. In this study, middle-aged workers reported poorer context-free mental health than younger and older workers did (Clark, Oswald, & Warr, 1996). However, unlike suppression of the curvilinear trend in Warr's (1992) analyses when covariates were added to the analyses, the curvilinear trend remains significant after adjustments for 80 control variables.

Job Satisfaction

Similar to evidence of age-related reductions in job stress and improvements in mental health, studies also show that aging is a protective factor for workers' job satisfaction. Remondet and Hansson's (1991) survey of white-collar workers, for example, found significantly higher levels of job satisfaction among older workers (54–72 years) than younger workers. More recently, the Conference Board (2007) reported a similar trend in a sample of 5,000 U.S. households. Nearly half of workers aged 55 years and older reported they are satisfied with their jobs—the largest satisfied proportion of any age group. Our analyses of 2004 HRS data extend this trend to very old workers in the U.S. (Sauter et. al., 2009). We found 28% of workers aged 51–64 years strongly agree that they "really enjoy" going to work. This strong level of agreement increased to 34% of workers aged 65–74 years and 46% of workers older than 74 years.

This trend toward age-related improvements in job satisfaction is further sustained in several large U.S., UK, and multinational studies. These implement more extensive controls for possible confounding dispositional factors (e.g., positive/negative affectivity and general mental health, work values and rewards), and job-related factors (e.g., salary, firm size, occupation, tenure, salary, supervisory status, working hours, and job autonomy) that might otherwise explain the age effect. Analyzing data from a sample of nearly 11,000 participants in the International Social Survey, Clark (2005) found age-related improvements in job satisfaction. Rode (2004) reported a similar trend in a longitudinal study of nearly 900 workers in the University of Michigan Americans' Changing Lives Survey. Our analyses of 2002 QWL data also revealed a significant, positive, linear relationship between age and job satisfaction (Sauter et al, 2009). Finally, a positive correlation between age and job satisfaction was also found in the Siu et al. (2001) study of Hong Kong managers. This effect, however, became nonsignificant when work-related explanatory variables were incorporated into the analyses.

Similar to findings in some of the studies of stress and mental health outcomes already described, several additional studies observed curvilinear relationships between age and job satisfaction that favor both younger and older workers. Using data from nearly 1,400 individuals participating in the 1972–1973 U.S. Quality of Employment Survey, Kalleberg and Loscocco (1983) first found a significant linear trend toward increased satisfaction among older workers, but they then uncovered significant curvilinear trends depicting reduced satisfaction in middle age. Clark et al. (1996) also found support for quadratic and linear effects of age in their analysis of the data from the 1991 British Household Panel Study. Job satisfaction levels decrease into the thirties, after which they pick up again and continue to increase into old age. The curvilinear trends observed in the Kalleberg and Loscocco (1983) and Clark et al. (1996) studies hold even with controls for numerous covariates in each study. Finally, a u-shaped relationship between age and job satisfaction was reported by Hochwarter, Ferris, Perrewé, Witt, and Kiewitz (2001) in a U.S. study of 2,200 university employees; here, satisfaction levels reached their lowest points for 40- to 49-year-old employees. This time, however, an additional linear trend was not found.

AGE DIFFERENCES IN JOB QUALITY

In comparison to the quantity of research on age and subjective well-being, studies of age differences in exposure to workplace risk factors for stress are relatively scarce. Of interest, findings from many of these studies are complementary to the results of investigations of age and subjective well-being and suggest improved job quality for older workers. Our own analyses of QWL data even provide evidence of higher-order effects of age, showing that aspects of the work environment are rated more positively by older and younger workers than by middle-aged workers. However, some studies are less encouraging, showing deterioration in various dimensions of job quality for older workers.

We begin with an overview of findings from the large European Survey of Working Conditions. Next, we draw comparisons of these findings with results from occupation-specific studies and other representative surveys of working populations. We then turn to results from our own analyses of the HRS and QWL. Finally, we report on QWL analyses that go beyond simple age–job quality associations to ask whether age moderates the relationship between job quality and subjective well being (i.e., the "differential sensitivity" effect raised in the introduction to this chapter).

Using data from the 2000 administration of the European Survey of Working Conditions, Ilmarinen (2005) and Molinié (2003) conducted comprehensive analyses of age differentials in the conditions of work. Results of these analyses suggest that age is generally protective with regard to exposure to stressful conditions. Workers over 45 years of age report greater opportunities to take breaks at will; increased control over their work tasks, work methods, and workloads; and stronger matches between their skills and job requirements. Additionally, these workers report reduced work pace, repetition of work, and shift work (although working hours were greater). One gender-specific effect worth noting is that older women report greater task complexity than younger women.

Several of the trends seen in the European Survey of Working Conditions, particularly between age and job control, replicate findings from earlier research. The Remondet and Hansson (1991) study of white-collar workers, for example, found that older workers reported fewer threats to job control, less disruption of performance, and greater job involvement levels. The study of Hong Kong managers by Siu et al. (2001) found older workers report a greater internal locus of work control and reduced total sources of stress than younger workers do. Similarly, data from Warr's

(1992) report on aging and well-being among British adults showed significant associations of age with job control (decision latitude) and demands. In view of the curvilinear functions seen in several studies of age and subjective well-being, it is interesting to note that only the quadratic form of the age term is significant in Warr's data. In this case, however, both control and demands are reduced for older (and younger) workers.

Evidence of age-related reductions in stressful working conditions measured in more general terms is also found in studies of aging and well-being in general populations. In a 1996 study of over 1,000 Boston males participating in the longitudinal Normative Aging Study (Aldwin, Sutton, Chiara, & Spiro, 1996), the prevalence of "work problems" declines steadily and substantially from the cohort aged 45–54 years to the older cohorts. Also, an Australian community study of nearly 7,500 individuals found significant reductions in reported crises at work from age 40–44 to age 60–64. There is also a reduction in threats to job loss from the age 20–24 to the age 60–64 cohort (Jorm, Windsor, Dear, Anstey, Christensen, & Rodgers, 2005).

Still, evidence of age-related deterioration in the work environment does appear in some of the literature. Several studies converge to suggest poorer supervisory interactions and reduced opportunities for development at work among older workers. Data from the European Survey of Working Conditions, for example, show that older workers face reductions in training and learning opportunities and fewer proactive and problem-solving discussions with supervisors (Ilmarinen, 2005). Warr and Birdi (1998) similarly found participation in voluntary development activities declines among older workers when studying 1,800 employees of a UK vehicle manufacturing company. Additionally, in a large representative sample of the Swedish working population, Aronsson, Gustafsson, and Dallner (2002) found reductions in supervisory support and encouragement for workers aged 46–55 years and reduced learning and development opportunities for workers aged 56–65 years.

Our own recent analyses of HRS and QWL data lend mixed support to the foregoing findings (Sauter et al., 2009). Similar to the reductions in job demands reported by Warr (1992), steady reductions across age strata in the 2004 HRS are seen in agreement with the statement that "the job requires me to do more difficult things than it used to." There was 49% agreement with this statement among 51–64 year old workers, compared to only 27% agreement among workers aged 64–74 years and 16% agreement of workers aged >74 years. Also, corresponding somewhat to the increasing control over rest breaks for older workers in the European Survey of Working Conditions (Illmarinen, 2005), HRS data show steady age-related increases in the proportion of workers reporting the ability to reduce their working hours, with 33% of workers aged 51–64 years, 54% of 64–74 years, and 60% of >74 years able to reduce their hours.

Our analyses of QWL data found age trends for eight of 23 job quality measures. All of these trends are favorable for older workers but one, and some consistency with other findings is evident. We found less work overload among older workers, which is similar to the age-related reductions in work demands reported by Warr (1992) and the reduced job difficulty seen in our analyses of the HRS. Our QWL analysis results also replicate Ilmarinen's (2005) findings of less exposure to shift work among older workers. Further, our QWL analyses showed reduced promotional opportunities among older workers, complementing findings of reduced developmental opportunities observed in earlier studies (Aronsson et al., 2002; Ilmarinen, 2005; Warr & Birdi, 1998).

Our analyses failed, however, to substantiate the associations of age with control or skill use that are rather prominent in earlier studies (Ilmarinen, 2005; Molinié, 2003; Remondet & Hansson, 1991; Sui et al., 2001, Warr, 1992). Also, we found several associations not evident in prior studies. We found that older workers report fewer long work days, fewer conflicting demands, fewer staffing problems, improved organizational climate, and improved job security. Some of the inconsistencies between our findings and other results may stem from differences in statistical approaches. While we employed multivariable statistical models in examining age-exposure relationships, simple descriptive analyses dominate the earlier studies. In fact, when simple bivariate analyses of QWL data were conducted, we found significant associations of age with both autonomy and skill use, which is similar to the associations of age with control and skill-match reported by Ilmarinen (2005). However, neither of these effects were significant in our final multiple regression models.

Finally, it is worth noting that all but the promotion, climate, and shift work effects in the QWL data are curvilinear, and the trend is consistent with effects for subjective well-being in some of the studies described earlier. Similar to the improvements in well-being seen in older and younger workers over that of middle-aged workers, relative improvements in working conditions were also evident among older and younger workers in the QWL sample.

As a last step in our analyses of the QWL, we investigated possible age differences in the effects of job quality factors. Prior research of this nature is sparse. The NRC (Wegman & McGee, 2004) uncovered a few relevant studies, but the results were mixed and inconclusive. Using multivariable statistical models once again, we investigated the effects of the interaction of age with 23 different job quality factors on nine health and well-being outcomes. The results of this effort, however, were limited and clustered around just a few exposures. Advancing age is associated with progressive improvements in subjective well-being when the social environment is supportive (coworkers are helpful and express interest) and with progressive decline in health outcomes when the environment is unsupportive. The same pattern of age-related divergence in health was seen for good and poor organizational climates—advancing age is associated with progressive improvements in subjective well-being when the climate is good and with progressive decline when the climate is poor. However, an opposite age effect occurred with variations in compensation (salary and benefit levels). Poor levels of compensation are associated with poorer health and subjective well-being for younger more so than older workers, and this age difference diminishes as compensation improves.

Some of these interactions might suggest that older workers have a heightened sensitivity to variations in job quality. However, other interpretations are possible. Because our analyses cannot untangle the effects of age and exposure history, it is possible that some of these effects result instead from the influence of cumulative exposure. The more favorable outcomes for older workers when the climate and social environment are positive, for example, could simply reflect the effects of older workers' longer exposures to positive work environments. Similarly, less favorable outcomes for older workers in the presence of a negative environment might reflect effects of longer exposure to these conditions for older workers.

DISCUSSION

Taken at face value, findings from research on the subjective well-being and job quality of older workers are encouraging. In general, the evidence points to reduced levels of job stress among older workers. There is also stronger evidence of improvements in the mental health and job satisfaction of older workers. Further, apart from findings of restricted developmental opportunities, exposures to job risk factors for stress appear to be no greater for older workers; in fact, they may even possibly be less than those for younger workers in some respects. There is some convergence of evidence suggesting, for example, that older workers experience improvements in job control, reductions in workload, and less exposure to shiftwork than their younger counterparts do. Finally, our recent analyses of QWL data provide little evidence that older workers are more vulnerable than younger workers to stressful workplace exposures.

Some of the age trends revealed in the present overview also show up in the results of a recent meta-analysis of 203 studies, where the relationship of age, occupational stressors, and outcomes was examined (Adams & Burns, 2008). Consistent with the age trends in subjective well-being summarized in this overview, this meta-analysis found modest negative correlations of age with depression and job dissatisfaction. Also, similar to the increase in job complexity among women workers reported by Ilmarinen (2005) and evidence of age-related reductions in demands and job difficulty in several studies (Ilmarinen, 2005; Warr, 1992; our HRS analyses), the Adams and Burns' meta-analysis found a modest positive correlation of age with job complexity and a negative association of age with role overload. In most cases, the confidence intervals for these correlations and other age effects uncovered in their meta-analysis crossed the zero point, suggesting a high degree of variability in the results of the examined studies and detracting from the significance of the observed relationships.

Various explanations have been offered for age-related improvements in the subjective well-being of workers, and many of these explanations apply as well to evidence of improved job quality among older workers, albeit more equivocally. Perhaps the most simple and straightforward explanation is that some of these trends may reflect the promotion or migration of older workers to better or higher-valued jobs and to positions that provide access to resources to better manage job demands (Warr, 1994; Wright & Hamilton, 1978). Curvilinear effects depicting a decline in well-being and job quality in the middle years in some study findings might result from the customary increases in occupational pressures in the midlife (Folkman, Lazarus, Pimley, & Novacek, 1987; Warr, 2007).

Other explanations focus on the contribution of psychological mechanisms to age trends in the subjective well-being of workers. Older or more senior workers may possess improved coping skills, improved emotional regulation, and better access to sources of support. Any or all of these potentially increase their capacities to deal with the pressures of work (Barnes-Farrell, 2005; Folkman et al., 1987; Hansson, Robson, & Limas, 2001; Warr, 1994). Along this line, changes in work-related aspirations and values of older workers, either as a coping mechanism or as a developmental process, may account in part for age differentials in the subjective well-being of workers. The salience of working conditions that are troublesome to younger workers may, for example, be reduced for older workers (Clark et al., 1996; Kalleberg & Loscocco, 1993; Warr, 2007). Some support for this viewpoint comes from a Finnish study comparing workers' ratings of workplace quality (mainly physical attributes) with the research team's independent ratings (Räsänen, Laitinen, & Rasa, 1997). The study found younger and older workers rate their work environments more satisfactorily than middle-aged workers do, but this trend is less evident in the researchers' ratings. The study concluded that "the younger workers' assessments were more realistic... whereas the other age groups seemed to be oversatisfied compared to the real situation" (Räsänen et al., 1997, p. 518).

Semmer and Schallenberger (1996) bring these two lines of reasoning—focus on the job and focus on workers' skills, capacities, and psychological adjustment—together into a more integrative framework to help explain the improved subjective well-being among older workers. They suggest, for example, that workers become more satisfied while growing older through a process of reciprocal adaptation, in which they personally develop in accordance with the demands of the job and concurrently mold the job to fit their own characteristics.

It is also possible that age-related improvements in the subjective well-being of workers originate in part from non-occupational experiences—namely, as a form of spillover from age-related improvements in context-free subjective well-being (Clark et al., 1996; Warr, 1997). Similar to observations in occupational samples, numerous studies employing community samples (i.e., samples including non-workers) have demonstrated age-related reductions in depression and anxiety (e.g., Christensen et al., 1999; Jorm et al., 2005; Regier et al., 1993), improvements in general mental health (Clark et al., 1996; Warr, 1997), reductions in stress (Aldwin et al., 1996), improvements in happiness (Diener & Suh, 1998; Yang, 2008), and improvements in life satisfaction (Mroczek & Spiro, 2005). Supporting this spillover hypothesis, many of these studies show worsening well-being through the middle years with improvement thereafter. This is similar to the curvilinear trends in well-being we described for many of the studies of occupation-specific samples.

Finally, it is possible that the favorable age trends reported in this chapter are in whole or part artifacts resulting from "healthy worker" effects or cohort effects that go undetected in the cross-sectional studies predominating in the literature presented here. Although labor force participation rates for older workers have been increasing for two decades, these rates (2005 estimates) still fall dramatically as workers age—dropping from 83% for workers 25–54 years old, to 63% for workers 55–64 years old, and to just 22% for workers 65–74 years old (Toosi, 2006). To the extent that declining health or low quality jobs contribute to early withdrawal from the labor force, it is possible that the favorable age trends described in this overview are biased by the presence of a surviving pool of workers who are uncharacteristically healthy or occupy uncharacteristically high-quality jobs. On the other hand, the u-shaped relationships between age and several of the job quality measures found in our analyses of QWL data show improvements in job quality in midlife (ages 40–50 years) when labor force participation rates are still highly stable, suggesting that healthy worker effects alone are insufficient explanations for these trends.

It is also possible that age-related trends reported in cross-sectional studies reflect differences between generations of workers in terms of the underlying conditions responsible for their well-being and not the effects of chronological aging. Warr (2007) comments, however, that a cohort effect is less plausible in view of the curvilinear relationships commonly reported between age and well-being. It would require a change in the underlying conditions from the oldest cohort (with higher levels of well-being) to the middle-age cohort (with lower levels of well-being), with a change back for the youngest cohort (with higher levels of well-being). Also relevant to concerns about cohort effects, Yang (2008) directly investigated cohort effects in a study of age and happiness using GSS data from 1972 to 2004. Of interest, results of this study showed that even after controlling for cohort effects, a gradient reflecting age-related increases in happiness is still evident.

In sum, the weight of the evidence would seem to suggest that work experiences are no more stressful for older persons than they are for younger workers. Taken together, findings for indicators of subjective well-being suggest even greater contentment among older workers, although evidence of improved job quality is more equivocal. While this trend is encouraging from the standpoint of protecting the health and safety of older workers and preserving their participation in the workforce, the literature on stress outcomes and job quality is not as well-developed, as the research on mental health and job satisfaction and the findings are somewhat uneven. Further research would be useful to better characterize these trends and untangle the contributing factors, but it is unlikely that much progress can be made in the absence of longitudinal panel studies or surveillance systems that capture data on job exposures and worker well-being across stages of the working life. Notably, this is the number one recommendation of the NRC for research to better understand the health and safety needs of older workers (Wegman & McGee, 2004).

We caution readers against over-generalizing the findings and trends revealed in this overview. Our focus was limited to the domain of subjective well-being (affective states) and occupational exposures most commonly associated with these types of outcomes. It is plausible, even perhaps likely, that age effects for other types of occupational health outcomes and exposures differ from trends reported here. For example, QWL analyses by Grosch and Pransky (2009) found a slight decline in back pain among older workers, which is similar to the age-related improvements in subjective well-being we have described here. However, they also found that physically demanding work (repetitive lifting) increases the risk of back pain considerably more for older workers than it does for younger workers (i.e., evidence of the vulnerability effect). This finding is very unlike our analyses of QWL data, which provided little evidence that poor job quality affects the well-being of older and younger workers differently.

NOTE

1. The findings and conclusions in this report are those of the authors and do not necessarily represent the views of the National Institute for Occupational Safety and Health.

REFERENCES

Adams, G. A., & Burns, G. N. (2008, March). *A meta-analysis of the relationship of age to occupational stressors and strains.* Poster presented at the APA/NIOSH Work, Stress, and Health conference, Washington, DC.

Aldwin, C. M., Sutton, K. J., Chiara, G., & Spiro, A. III. (1996). Age differences in stress, coping, and appraisal: Findings from the normative aging study. *Journal of Gerontology: Psychological Sciences, 51B*(4), 179–188.

Aronsson, G., Gustafsson, K., & Dallner, M. (2002). Work environment and health in different types of temporary jobs. *European Journal of Work and Organizational Psychology, 11*(2), 151–175.

Barnes-Farrell, J. L. (2005). Older workers. In J. Barling, K. Kelloway, & M. Frone (Eds.), *Handbook of work stress* (pp. 431–454). Thousand Oaks, CA: Sage Press.

Blackmore, E. R., Stansfeld, S. A., Weller, I., Munce, S., Zagorski, B. M., & Stewart, D. E. (2007). Major depressive episodes and work stress: Results from a national population survey. *American Journal of Public Health, 97*(11), 1—6.

Centers for Disease Control and Prevention. (CDC). (2000). *Measuring healthy days.* Atlanta, GA: Author.

Christensen, H., Jorm, A. F., MacKinnon, A. J., Korten, A. E., Jacomb, P. A., Henderson, A. S., & Rodgers, B. (1999). Age differences in depression and anxiety symptoms: A structural equation modeling analysis of data from a general population sample. *Psychological Medicine, 29,* 325–339.

Clark, A. E. (2005). Your money or your life: Changing job quality in OECD countries. *British Journal of Industrial Relations, 43*(3), 377–400.

Clark, A., Oswald, A., & Warr, P. (1996). Is job satisfaction U-shaped in age? *Journal of Occupational and Organizational Psychology, 69,* 57–81.

Conference Board. (2007, February). *US job satisfaction declines.* Retrieved from http://www.conference-board.org

Davis, J. A., Smith, T. W., & Marsden, P. V. (2002). *General social surveys, 1972–2002: Cumulative codebook* (NORC Ed.). Chicago, IL: National Opinion Research Center.

Diener, E., & Suh, E. M. (1998). Subjective well-being and age: An international analysis. *Annual Review of Gerontology and Geriatrics, 17,* 304–324.

Elovainio, M., Forma, P., Kivimäki, M., Sinervo, T., Sutinen, R., & Laine, M. (2005). Job demands and job control as correlates of early retirement thoughts in Finnish social and health care employees. *Work and Stress, 19*(1), 84–92.

Folkman, S., Lazarus, R. S., Pimley, S., & Novacek, J. (1987). Age differences in stress and coping processes. *Psychology and Aging, 2*(2), 171–184.

Frone, M. R., Russell, M., & Barnes, G. M. (1996). Work–family conflict, gender, and health-related outcomes: A study of employed parents in two community samples. *Journal of Occupational Health Psychology, 1*(1), 57–69.

Griffiths, A. (2007). Healthy work for older workers: Work design and management factors. In W. Loretto, S. Vickerstaff, & P. White (Eds.), *The future for older workers: New perspective* (pp. 125–141). Bristol, UK: Policy Press.

Griffiths, A., Knight, A., & Mohd Mahudin, N.D. (2009). *Ageing, work-related stress, and health: Reviewing the evidence.* London, UK: Help the Aged.

Grosch, J. W., & Pransky, G. S. (2009). Safety and health issues for an aging workforce. In S. Czaja & J. Sharit (Eds.), *The future of work for an aging population* (pp. 334–358). Baltimore, MD: Johns Hopkins Press.

Hansson, R. O., Robson, S. M., & Limas, M. J. (2001). Stress and coping among older workers. *Work, 17,* 247–256.

Hennekens, K., & Tazelaar, F. (1994). Early retirement of civil servants in the Netherlands. *Journal of Applied Social Psychology,* 24, 1927–1943.

Hilton, M. F., Whiteford, H. A., Sheridan, J. S., Cleary, C. M., Chant, D. C., Wang, P. S., & Kessler, R. C. (2008). The prevalence of psychological distress in employees and associated occupational risk factors. *Journal of Occupational and Environmental Medicine, 50*(7), 746–757.

Hochwarter, W. A., Ferris, G. R., Perrewé, P. L., Witt, L. A., & Kiewitz, C. (2001). A note on the nonlinearity of the age–job-satisfaction relationship. *Journal of Applied Social Psychology, 31*(6), 1223–1237.

Ilmarinen, J. (2005). *Towards a longer worklife! Ageing and the quality of worklife in the European Union.* Helsinki, Finland: Finnish Institute of Occupational Health.

Jorm, A. F., Windsor, T. D., Dear, K. B. G., Anstey, K. J., Christensen, H., & Rodgers, B. (2005). Age group differences in psychological distress: The role of psychosocial risk factors that vary with age. *Psychological Medicine,* 35, 1253–1263

Kalleberg, A. L., & Loscocco, K. A. (1983). Aging, values, and rewards: Explaining age differences in job satisfaction. *American Sociological Review, 48*(1), 78–90.

Kowalski-Trakofler, K. M., Steiner, L. J., and Schwerha, D. J. (2005). Safety considerations for the aging workforce. *Safety Science, 43,* 779–793.

Mein, G., Martikainen, P., Stansfeld., S. S., Brunner, E. J., Fuhrer, R., & Marmot, M.G. (2000). Predictors of early retirement in British civil servants. *Age and Aging, 29,* 529–536.

Molinié, A.-F. (2003). Age and working conditions in the European Union. Ireland: European Foundation for the improvement of Living and Working Conditions. Retrieved from http://www.eurofound.eu.int/publications/files/EF02107EN.pdf

Mosisa A., & Hipple, S. (2006). Trends in labor force participation in the United States. *Monthly Labor Review, 129*(10), 35–57.

Mroczek, D. K., & Spiro, A. (2005). Change in life satisfaction during adulthood: Findings from the Veterans Affairs Normative Aging Study. *Journal of Personality and Social Psychology, 88,* 189–202.

Räsänen, T., Laitenen, H., & Rasa, P-L. (1997). The effect of age on subjective assessment of work environment. In P. Seppäla, T. Luopajärvi, C-H. Nygård, & M. Mattila (Eds.), *Proceedings of the 13th Triennial Congress of the International Ergonomics Association: Vol 5. From Experience to Innovation* (pp. 516–518). Helsinki, Finland: Finnish Institute of Occupational Health.

Regier, D. A., Farmer, M. E., Rae, D. S., Myers, J. K., Kramer, M., Robins, L. N.,... Locke, B. Z. (1993). One-month prevalence of mental disorders in the United States and sociodemographic characteristics: The Epidemiologic Catchment Area study. *Acta Psychiatrica Scandinavia,* 88, 35–47.

Remondet, J. H., & Hansson, R. O. (1991). Job-related threats to control among older employees. *Journal of Social Issues, 47*(4), 129–141.

Rode, J. C. (2004). Job satisfaction and life satisfaction revisited: A longitudinal test of an integrated model. *Human Relations, 57*(9), 1205–1230.

Robertson, A., & Tracy, C. S. (1998). Health and productivity of older workers. *Scandinavian Journal of Work, Environment, & Health,* 24(2), 85–97.

Sauter, S. L., Streit, J. M., & Hanseman, D. J. (2009). Work organization and health in an aging workforce: Observations from the NIOSH Quality of Work Life Survey. In S. Czaja, S. & J. Sharit (Eds.), *The future of work for an aging population* (pp. 359–393). Baltimore, MD: Johns Hopkins Press.

Semmer, N., & Schallberger, U. (1996). Selection, socialization, and mutual adaptation: Resolving discrepancies between people and work. *Applied Psychology: An International Review, 45*(3), 263–288.

Siegreist, J., Wahrendorf, M., von dem Knesebeck, O., Jürges, H., & Börsch-Supan, A. (2006). Quality of work, well-being, and intended early retirement of older employees—Baseline results from the SHARE study. *The European Journal of Public Health, 17*(1), 62–68.

Siu, O., Spector, P. E., Cooper, C. L., & Donald, I. (2001). Age differences in coping and locus of control: A study of managerial stress in Hong Kong. *Psychology and Aging, 16*(4), 707–710.

Smith, A. (2001). Perceptions of stress at work. *Human Resource Management Journal, 11,* 74–86.

Swanson, V., Power, K., & Simpson, R. (1996). A comparison of stress and job satisfaction in females and male GPs and consultants. *Stress Medicine, 12,* 17–26.

Toosi, M. (2006). A new look at long-term labor force projections to 2050. *Monthly Labor Review, 129*(11), 19–39.

Tuomi, K., Ilmarinen, J., Martikainen, R., Aalto, L., & Klockars, M. (1997). Aging, work, life-style and work ability among Finnish municipal workers in 1981–1992. *Scandinavian Journal of Work Environment and Health, 23*(suppl. 1), 58–65.

Tuomi, K., Ilmarinen, J., Seitsamo, J., Huuhtanen, P., Martikaininen, R., Nygård, C., & Klockars, M. (1997). Summary of the Finnish research project (1981-1992) to promote the health and work ability of aging workers. *Scandinavian Journal of Work Environment and Health, 23*(suppl. 1), 66–71.

Warr, P. (1992). Age and occupational well-being. *Psychology and Aging,* 7(1), 37–45.

Warr, P. (1994). Age and employment. In H. C. Triandis, M. D. Dunnette, & L. M. Hough, eds., *Handbook of industrial and organizational psychology* (Vol. 4, pp. 485–550). Palo Alto, CA: Consulting Psychologists Press.

Warr, P. B. (1997). Age, work, and mental health. In K. W. Schaie & C. Schooler (Eds.), *The impact of work on older adults* (pp. 252–296). New York, NY: Springer.

Warr, P. (2007). *Work, happiness, and unhappiness.* Mahwah, NJ: Lawrence Erlbaum Associates.

Warr, P. & Birdi, K. (1998). Employee age and voluntary development activity. *International Journal of Training and Development, 2*(3), 190–204.

Wegman, D. H., & McGee, J. P. (Eds.). (2004). *Health and safety needs of older workers.* National Research Council and the Institute of Medicine, Committee on the Health and Safety Needs of Older Workers. Division of Behavioral and Social Sciences and Education. Washington, DC: The National Academies Press.

Williams, S., & Cooper, C. L. (1996). *Occupational Stress Indicator Version 2.* Harrogate, North Yorkshire, UK: RAD Ltd.

Wright, J. D., & Hamilton, R. F. (1978). Work satisfaction and age: Some evidence for the "job change" hypothesis. *Social Forces, 56,* 1140–1158.

Yang, Y. (2008). Social inequalities in happiness in the United States, 1972–2004: An age-period-cohort analysis. *American Sociological Review, 73,* 204–226.

SECTION II

EXAMINING IMBALANCE AND MISMATCH MODELS OF STRESS

CHAPTER 5

SOCIAL REWARD AND HEALTH

How to Reduce Stress at Work and Beyond[1]

Johannes Siegrist
University of Duesseldorf

It is obvious that the nature of work has undergone rather fundamental changes in economically advanced societies. Industrial mass production no longer dominates the labor market. This is due, in part, to technological progress, and in part to a growing number of jobs available in the service sector. Many jobs are confined to information processing, controlling, and coordination. Sedentary rather than physically strenuous work is becoming more and more dominant. Moreover, the traditional separation of the spheres of work and home is vanishing. Homework, participation in virtual networks, and an unprecedented degree of flexibility in local and temporal work arrangements contribute to this process. Traditional continuous occupational careers are increasingly being replaced by job change, fix-term contract, temporary work, or self-employment. With the advent of econom-

Coping and Prevention, pages 75–91

ic globalization, pressure towards an increase in return on investment has been growing over the past two decades. As a consequence, work pressure increased considerably in private, and increasingly in public sectors, due to financial cuts (Ostry & Spiegel, 2004). Another consequence of economic globalization concerns the segmentation of the labor market, a related increase in income inequality, and a substantial loss of jobs. A large part of the workforce in advanced societies suffers from job insecurity, low wages and salaries, and a low level of safety at work. With the globalization of labor markets, competition among employees has been increasing, and a growing proportion of workers have been exposed to mergers, downsizing, outsourcing, or redundancy (Landsbergis 2003).

These changes are not confined to the most economically advanced societies, but are now spreading across rapidly developing countries, such as Brazil in Latin America or India, China, and Vietnam in Asia (Schnall, Dobson, & Rosskam, 2009). Globalization, if adequately managed, can contribute to a rise in living standard, economic growth, and gain in population health. However, growing socioeconomic inequalities and adverse working and employment conditions are likely to afflict the health of working populations. Therefore, it is important to identify major determinants of the work-related burden of disease and to strengthen interventions with the aim of reducing this burden and promoting healthy work.

In this chapter the focus is restricted to the analysis of a stressful psychosocial work environment, its documented effects on physical and mental health, and the role of stress management in reducing the burden of work-related disease where different levels of intervention (personal, interpersonal, organization-related, policy-related) are considered. Thus, important areas of scientific evidence and practical intervention—such as occupational safety including injury prevention, traditional occupational medicine dealing with toxic components of work places and work environments, and temporal aspects of work organization (mainly shift work)—are not considered. Yet, ideally, these relatively well-established fields of knowledge and occupational health practice are to be incorporated into more comprehensive approaches that deal with new challenges of work and employment, as mentioned above.

How can we define and measure a stressful psychosocial environment? Is it possible to separate the environmental or situational components from the personal components of individual workers, or do we need transactional approaches that combine situational and personal characteristics? How can we establish scientific evidence on links between stressful work and elevated health risks of exposed workers? These questions require updated answers, reflecting the current state of scientific developments. But again, as this field of research is rapidly expanding, thus preventing a balanced overview on a few pages, a selective answer is given, focusing on an approach that has received growing attention in international occupational health research in the recent past: the role of social reward at work. The theoretical basis and the measurement of this approach are outlined in the next section.

SOCIAL REWARD AND STRESS: THEORETICAL BASIS

In general terms, a stressor is defined as a challenge that taxes or threatens an exposed person due to her limited capability of successfully coping with it. In the context of work and employment, psychosocial stressors often become manifest as recurrent demands, threats, or conflicts that cannot be disregarded or escaped, but require active coping efforts. Whether a psychosocial stressor at work elicits significant stress reactions in the organism of the exposed person depends on its quality and intensity, as well as on the coping ability and available resources of the person. Thus, the stress process is basically a transactional process involving characteristics of the work and employment situation (organizational features) and characteristics of the working people (capabilities, resources).

What is the link between social reward and stress? Why is social reward, or more exactly its lack or its inappropriate experience at work, a psychosocial stressor? To answer these questions it is important to consider some of the basic contributions of work and employment to human functioning and well-being. In advanced societies, having a job is most often a prerequisite for a continuous income and, more so than any other social circumstance, employment characteristics determine adult socioeconomic status. Beyond economic livelihood, a person's occupation is an important aim of long-term socialization, thus providing opportunities for personal growth and development. In addition, working in an organization enables people to participate in social networks beyond primary groups. The need for positive self-experience is intimately linked to these functions of work. Having a secure job, being adequately paid, being able to meet challenging demands and to get favorable feedback, developing skills, and being supported by colleagues are important prerequisites for positive self-experience, functioning, and well-being at work. Positive self-experience manifests itself mainly through recurrent feelings of self-efficacy and self-esteem.

Self-efficacy, the belief of a person in her ability to accomplish tasks, is based on a favorable evaluation of one's competence and of expected outcomes, strengthening the experience of personal control. Self-esteem, the continued sense of a person's positive self-worth, is based on esteem and appreciation expressed by significant others, strengthening the experience of social reward. Importantly, work and employment conditions that enable people to experience personal control and social reward are likely to favor well-being, health, and functioning, whereas conditions that prevent these experiences may trigger stress reactions and reduce working people's health and well-being in the long run. Solid scientific evidence is now available that demonstrates the afflictions of recurrent loss or lack of personal control to the human organism (Henry & Stephens, 1977; McEwen, 1998), mainly by excessive arousal of distinct stress axes linking brain and autonomic nervous system activity with peripheral organ systems (Weiner, 1992). Similarly, loss or frustration of relevant social rewards was shown to impair the brain reward circuitry, an essential trigger of human motivation, and to elicit long-lasting stress reactions including susceptibility to addiction (Schultz, Dayan, & Montague, 1997).

Given these strong links of experiencing personal control and social reward with remaining healthy and well it is crucial to identify those work and employment conditions that prevent these experiences and, by doing so, act as psychosocial stressors that elicit recurrent stress reactions in exposed working people. Two theoretical models of stressful work have been developed in this frame: the demand–control model and the effort–reward imbalance model. The demand–control model (Karasek & Theorell, 1990) posits that stressful experience at work results from a distinct job task profile defined by two dimensions, the psychological demands put on the working person and the degree of control or decision latitude available to the person to perform the required tasks. Jobs defined by high demands in combination with low control are stressful because they limit the individual's autonomy and sense of control while generating continued pressure ("high job strain"). A third dimension, social support at work, was added to the original formulation. In this formulation, the highest level of strain would be expected in jobs that are characterized by high demand, low control, and low social support at work or social isolation ("iso-strain jobs") (Johnson & Hall, 1988).

While this model is focused on specific workplace characteristics without considering personal characteristics of the working person, the second model to some extent takes personal coping characteristics into account. Moreover, this model, effort-reward imbalance, is concerned with stressful features of the work contract rather than of the job task (Siegrist 1996). This model builds on the notion of social reciprocity, a fundamental principle of all types of transactions that are characterized by some form of utility. Social reciprocity lies at the core of the work contract which defines distinct obligations or tasks to be performed in exchange with adequate rewards. These rewards include money, esteem and career opportunities (promotion, job security). Contractual reciprocity operates through norms of return expectancy, where effort spent by employees is reciprocated by equitable rewards from employers (see Figure 5.1). The effort–reward imbalance model claims that lack of reciprocity occurs frequently under

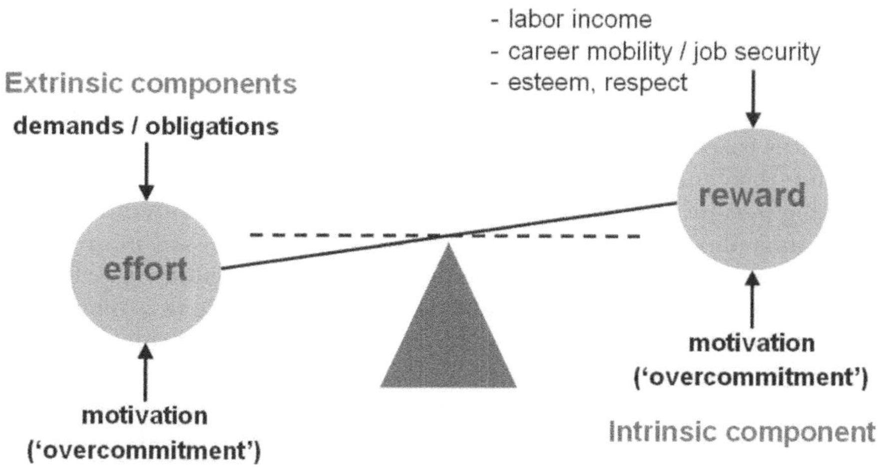

Figure 5.1 The model of effort-reward imbalance at work (modified from Siegrist, 1996).

specific conditions. Failed reciprocity, in terms of high cost and low gain, elicits strong negative emotions and associated stress reactions with adverse long-term health consequences. "High cost–low gain" conditions at work occur frequently if employed people have no alternative choice in the labor market (e.g., due to low qualification) or if they make strategic choices to spend additional efforts in order to improve their career prospects in highly competitive professions. Moreover, there are psychological reasons for a recurrent mismatch between efforts and reward at work. People characterized by a motivational pattern of excessive work-related overcommitment may strive towards continuously high achievement because of their underlying need for approval and esteem at work. Although these excessive efforts often are not met by adequate rewards, overcommitted people tend to maintain their level of involvement.

In summary, the model of effort–reward imbalance at work maintains that people experiencing dependency, strategic choice and overcommitment, either separately or in combination, are often exposed to failed contractual reciprocity at work and its health-adverse consequences. The model combines organizational features with personal coping characteristics. The demand–control and the effort–reward imbalance models complement each other by focusing on "toxic" components of job task profiles and employment contracts respectively. Low control and low reward are assumed to be equally stressful experiences in the context of work that requires high levels of effort. They both elicit negative emotions and enhanced stress responses with adverse long-term health consequences.

METHODOLOGICAL APPROACH

Several methodological approaches to the study of psychosocial stress at work and its effects on health were developed. These include objective measures based on observational data from trained experts or on administrative data and standardized questionnaires based on self-reports from working persons, assessed at individual or aggregate level. Advantages and disadvantages of each measurement approach are discussed in great detail among scientists, but cannot be detailed here (Rau, Morling, & Rösler, 2010). There are at least three reasons that justify the use of psychometrically validated self-assessed questionnaires in research on work stress and health, as defined by the demand–control (support) model (Karasek, Brisson, Kawakami, Houtman, Bongers, & Amick, 1998) and the effort–reward imbalance model (Leineweber et al., 2010; Siegrist et al., 2004). First, it is difficult to assess some of these dimensions in terms of direct observation of work places (e.g., degree of social support at work, esteem or appreciation from superiors or colleagues) or by relying on administrative data. In addition, issues of inter-rater reliability, logistic and economic aspects of data collection need to be considered. Second, according to basic stress-theoretical notions, the individual experience of an adverse psychosocial work environment triggers emotional and autonomic nervous system responses and, thus, can act as a proxy measure of the respective exposure. Clearly, potential measurement error must be considered a challenge that may be minimized by adjusting for reporting style and specific personality characteristics of respondents. Third, given the fact that prospective cohort studies based on large samples are needed to test causal associations of work stress with incident disease, standardized questionnaires are an economic and feasible approach to assessing exposures.

Effort–reward imbalance (ERI) at work is measured by a standardized, psychometrically validated self-report questionnaire containing the three scales "effort" (6 items), "reward" (11 items that represent the three dimensions of financial and career-related rewards, of esteem and of job security in respective subscales), and "overcommitment" (6 items representing the intrinsic model component). The Likert-scaled items are rated by respondents, and a sum score of each scale is calculated. Psychometric properties of these scales were extensively assessed, including internal consistency, discriminant and criterion validity, sensitivity to change, and factorial invariance (de Jonge, van der Linden, Schaufeli, Peter, & Siegrist, 2008). Moreover, confirmatory factor analysis revealed three moderately correlated second-order factors ("effort," "reward," "overcommitment," where "reward" is further specified into three theoretically relevant subcomponents) loading on a general third factor that represents the latent (theoretical) construct. Based on these premises, a short version containing 16 instead of 23 items was developed more recently, again documenting satisfactory psychometric properties (Leineweber et al., 2010; Siegrist et al., 2009).Both versions are available in a number of languages, including English (Siegrist et al., 2004) and Portuguese-Brazilian (Griep et al. 2009).

In epidemiological studies it is often convenient to represent the independent variable in terms of a single binary or continuous measure. Therefore, a ratio of the two variables "effort" and "reward" was constructed to represent the core theoretical notion in a quantitative way, with a possible cut-point of 1.0 representing a balance between efforts and rewards, and higher values representing the risk condition (Siegrist et al., 2004). Quantitative self-report data have received methodological criticisms given their limited validity. Yet, despite obvious limitations, satisfying correlations with more objective measures and with computerized ambulatory diaries were reported (Johnston, Beedie, & Jones, 2006; Tsutsumi, Nagami, Morimoto, & Matoba, 2002). It should also be noted that in a stress-theoretical perspective, subjective appraisals are an important source of information when estimating their potential emotional and psychobiological impact.

Given the advantage of a short, standardized quantitative measure with comparable scores the ERI questionnaire has been applied in a large number of prospective epidemiological studies, cross-sectional, case-control, and experimental including intervention studies. Study populations include industrial and service sectors, both gender and all age groups, and participants from Western industrialized societies as well as from rapidly developing societies (for reviews see Siegrist, 2009; Tsutsumi & Kawakami, 2004; van Vegchel, de Jonge, Bosma, & Schaufeli, 2005). The next section gives a selective review of major empirical evidence linking effort–reward imbalance at work with poor health and elevated risks of stress-related physical and mental disorders, including some information on psychobiological and behavioral pathways.

EMPIRICAL EVIDENCE

The relatively strongest evidence on associations of psychosocial stress at work in terms of low social reward compare to efforts spent with poor health is obtained from prospective epidemiological observational studies. This is due to the temporal sequence (exposure assessment precedes disease onset), the usual sample size (based on statistical power calculation and allowing for adjustment for confounding variables in multivariate analysis), and the quantification of subsequent disease risk following exposure (odds ratio of disease in exposed vs. non exposed individuals). Additional evidence comes from case-control studies, cross-sectional studies, ambulatory monitoring studies, and experimental or quasi-experimental investigations including intervention trials. All these types of study designs were applied to analyze associations of ERI with stress-related disorders and their pathways.

Prospective Epidemiological Studies

The majority of prospective investigations using social reward deficiency (i.e., effort–reward imbalance at work) as a predictor of stress-related disorders were concerned with coronary heart disease or depression. This choice is well justified in view of their contribution to the global burden of disease. By the year 2020, depression and coronary heart disease will be the leading causes of premature death and of life years defined by disability worldwide (Mathers, Lopez, & Murray, 2006). Evidence of elevated risks of coronary heart disease among exposed versus non-exposed employees was found in two blue-collar populations in Germany (Siegrist, Peter, Junge, Cremer, & Seidel, 1990) and in Finland (Kivimäki, Leino-Arjas, Luukonen, Riihimäki, Vahtera, & Kirjonen, 2002), and in the Whitehall II study of British civil servants (Bosma, Peter, Siegrist, & Marmot, 1998; Kuper, Singh-Manoux, Siegrist, & Marmot, 2002). Findings of a further prospective study are in line with the model's assumption, although they are based on crude operational measures (Lynch, Krause, Kaplan, Tuomilehto, & Salonen, 1997). One report was negative (for review, see Eller et al., 2009; Kivimäki, Virtanen, Elovainio, Kouvonen, Väänänen, & Vahtera, 2006). Overall, a relative risk of about 1.8 is observed in employees with social reward deficiency at work, after adjusting for relevant confounders. Results are more consistent among men than women, and more so in middle-aged than in older aged populations. Even if the reported odds ratio or relative risk is not large, effects in absolute terms are considerable, given the fact that between 10 and 25% of the samples were exposed to work stress in terms of this model.

Further findings from several studies are now available with regard to depression, either diagnosed by physicians or defined on the basis of clinically validated self-administered questionnaires. Results from studies examining associations of ERI with depression are based on large samples covering several ten thousand working men and women from 12 European countries. Overall, the relative risk of developing depression or relevant depressive symptoms is twice as high among those scoring high on ERI scales (high effort, low reward, high overcommitment; for review Siegrist & Dragano 2008). Additional health outcomes of prospective studies testing the ERI model are type 2 diabetes, alcohol dependence and sleep disturbances (where significant effects are restricted to men), poor physical and mental functioning, and poor self-rated health (for review, see Siegrist, 2009). Moreover, risks of musculoskeletal pain (Krause et al., 2009) and of sickness absence (Ala-Mursala et al., 2005; Head et al., 2007) were elevated as a function of reward frustration at work. Despite their methodological strengths, prospective epidemiological investigations provide little insight into the pathways underlying the observed statistical observations. Therefore, supplementary information is needed (see following section).

Studies of Pathways and Interventions

Two pathways are generally studied in research on work stress and health: the mediation of effects by health-adverse behaviors, such as smoking, poor health, or lack of physical exercise, and the mediation by chronic bodily stress reactions triggering "allostatic load" via psychobiological mechanisms and resulting ultimately in structural lesions and adaptive breakdown (McEwen, 1998). Here, this latter pathway is discussed in some detail, as the behavioral pathways have been reviewed elsewhere (Siegrist & Rödel, 2006).

Psychobiological processes are the pathways through which health-adverse psychosocial stressors activate autonomic, neuroendocrine, immune, and inflammatory responses via the organism's stress axes. Several studies were conducted so far testing effort–reward imbalance at work and its impact on cardiovascular, stress hormone, and immune parameters. Two such studies concern ambulatory blood pressure monitoring where overcommitted, low status men were shown to exhibit elevated systolic blood pressure throughout the workday (Steptoe, Siegrist, Kirschbaum, & Marmot, 2004) and where stressed healthy computer employees were shown to manifest elevated heart rate, systolic blood pressure, and a tendency towards reduced heart rate variability (Vrijkotte, van Doornen, & de Geus, 2000). Additional studies explored associations of ERI with secretion of stress hormones, e.g., cortisol, adrenalin and noradrenalin. A dysregulated secretion pattern was observed in a majority of these studies (Bellingrath, Weigl, & Kudielka, 2008; Hurwitz Eller, Netterstrom, & Hansen, 2006; Steptoe et al., 2004; Wirtz, Siegrist, Rimmele, & Ehlert, 2008). In view of the importance of inflammation for the development of cardiovascular disease and other stress-related disorders (Stansfeld & Marmot, 2002) an experimental study is of particular interest documenting higher concentrations of C-reactive protein (a marker of inflammation) following exposure to a standardized mental stress test in participants scoring high on ERI measures, compared to participants with less or no work stress (Hamer, Williams, Vuonovirta, Giacobazzi, Gibson, & Steptoe, 2006; see Figure 5.2).

More recently, in a group of teachers exposed to a standardized laboratory stressor (the Trier Social Stress Test), high effort in combination with low reward and high overcommitment were associated with lower levels of natural killer cells and with increased pro-inflammatory activity (Bellingrath et

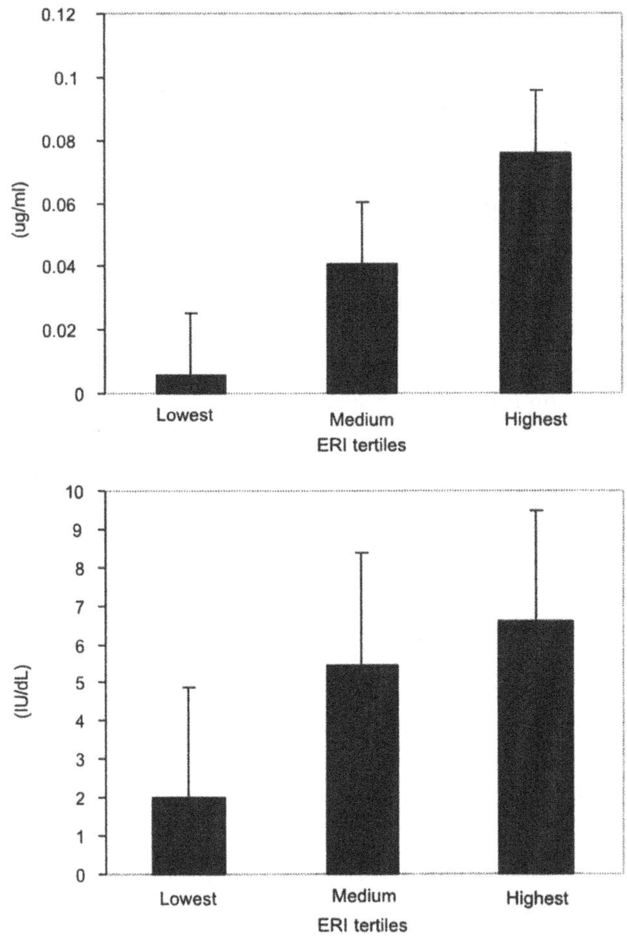

Figure 5.2 The effect of effort-reward imbalance at work (ERI tertiles) on C-reactive protein (upper part) and von Willebrand factor responses (lower part) to mental stress. Values are mean ± SEM adjusted for age, Body Mass Index, and baseline levels (n = 92 men aged 33.1 ± 8.6 years). *Source*: Hamer et al. (2006), reprinted by permission of the publisher.

al., 2010). Taken together, naturalistic and experimental studies supplement epidemiological evidence by demonstrating psychobiological processes that possibly mediate the observed associations of psychosocial adversity at work with stress-related disorders.

Up to now, few intervention studies only were conducted with explicit reference to the ERI model. One such study involved a 12-session stress management program among urban bus drivers where skills of coping with stressful work were improved, and where superiors were trained to appreciate the bus drivers' work more closely and to enhance communication and collaboration across hierarchies. Although no health measures were assessed as outcomes, mean scores of overcommitment, a stress-enhancing personal pattern of coping with work demands, were significantly reduced in the intervention as compared to the control group, and this effect persisted over months (Aust, Peter, & Siegrist, 1997). Another stress management intervention based on this model was conducted in a group of middle management employees of a large manufactoring plant in Germany. After one year, perceived stress reactivity decreased significantly in the intervention as compared to the control group, and a similar trend was observed for a biological stress marker, alpha-amylase (Limm et al., 2010). Finally, a quasi-experimental design with an intervention and a control group was applied among healthcare workers in Canadian hospitals. A participatory approach with an intervention team was implemented, aiming at a reduction of a health-adverse psychosocial work environment as defined by the demand–control–support and the effort–reward imbalance models (Bourbonnais, Brisson, Vinet, Vezina, & Lower, 2006). Three years after the intervention, the mean of all adverse work factors (except psychological demands) and the mean of all health indicators (in particular burnout) was significantly more favorable in the experimental than the control hospital, after adjusting for pre-intervention measures (Bourbonnais, Brisson, & Vezina, 2011). These findings provide promising preliminary evidence of feasibility and effectiveness of stress reduction at the organizational level.

IMPLICATIONS FOR STRESS MANAGEMENT AND FUTURE DIRECTIONS

There are at least four levels of intervention approaches aimed at reducing stress at work and its related burden of disease. The first three dimensions are directed to single organizations—companies, firms, or administrative units. Here, measures can target (1) individual persons—that is, single employees or groups of employees (individual level of stress management), (2) collaborating teams or managers and supervisors (interpersonal level of stress management, in particular leadership training), or (3) organizational units or total organizations in terms of work redesign, division of work, personnel development etc. (structural level of stress management). Under optimal conditions, these three dimensions are combined in order to produce intervention effects that are enhanced and sustainable. A fourth dimension concerns the level of national labor and social policies or even international regulations of employment and working conditions that protect workers' health. Although this dimension is not discussed in the current context, it is important to note that far-reaching effects can be produced by such policy interventions. For instance, in a recent comparative study in Europe, consistent associations were observed between the amount of investment in workers' unemployment protection or in workers' continuous education and training on one side and the quality of a health-conducive work environment on the other side (Dragano, Siegrist, & Wahrendorf, 2011). Moreover, the effect size of a nation's mean level of work stress (effort–reward imbalance, low control) on risk of reduced mental health (depressive symptoms) was relatively weakest in Scandinavian countries with an elaborated welfare policy and was relatively strongest in a liberal state—the United Kingdom—where employment protection was weak.

At the level of single companies or other types of organizations, available evidence indicates that stress management at individual and interpersonal levels produces more consistent and stronger effects on workers' health and well-being than structural measures of stress management, although research designs are generally weak and the number of studies addressing structural measures is low. Therefore, future structural interventions need to consider specific moderators of the effects of work-oriented interventions in order to improve outcomes. In this context, Biron, Cooper, and Bond (2009) emphasize the role of top management support and participatory processes, the availability of resources for sustainable implementation, a sound risk assessment at entry, an ongoing process valuation, and a well-grounded intervention approach.

Clearly, the work stress models discussed in this chapter offer options of identifying promising intervention targets. For instance, according to the demand–control model, job redesign in terms of job enrichment, task or work time control, and skill training are measures that already proved to produce beneficial effects (Landsbergis, 2009). Similarly, the ERI model proposes the provision of rewards that are proportionate to workers' efforts (e.g., compensatory wage systems, models of gain sharing), the implementation of non-monetary means of recognition and appreciation, and the establishment of fair procedures of career advancement (see above). Both models stress the critical role of leadership training, and a recent review of effects of leadership interventions on employees' well-being demonstrates a rich and elaborate range of training approaches and beneficial outcomes (Kelloway & Barling, 2010). By far the largest amount of evidence is currently available at the individual level of stress management. Respective programs may offer non-specific prevention measures, such as relaxation, spirituality (yoga), or art. Alternatively, cognitive behavioral or psychodynamic therapies may be applied that are modified according to theoretical orientations and practical purposes. It is important to stress that these latter interventions are particularly useful in secondary and tertiary prevention, specifically as an element of interventions that aim at reintegrating sick and disabled persons into work and employment (Black, 2008). Developing and implementing measures of work-related programs of stress management and health promotion at different levels is a policy measure of high priority. This conclusion is supported by available evidence of the work-stress related burden of disease and its costs to public health and the economy.

The model of effort–reward imbalance was preliminarily developed and tested in the context of work and employment. However, its relevance reaches beyond paid work as it reflects a basic stressful experience of social exchange, the frustration of fair reward expectancies of people who invested in this exchange. Therefore, future scientific and practical developments related to this model concern its application to unpaid work (e.g., voluntary work, homework, caring; see Wahrendorf , Ribet, Zins, Goldberg, & Siegrist, 2010), schoolwork (Li, Shang, Wang, & Siegrist, 2010), as well as close social relationships requiring investments which may be shared in unequal ways, such as in partnership or between parents and children (Chandola, Marmot, & Siegrist, 2007). Extending evidence on health-adverse effects of failed reciprocity in basic patterns of social exchange may contribute to the development of a society where fairness, equity and trust matter more than selfish attitudes and behaviors.

In this chapter, a selective view of this far-reaching topic of health-adverse work environments was given, by focusing in more detail on one specific aspect, the deleterious effects on health produced by inappropriate or missing rewards at work. Even such a restricted, focused approach demonstrates the far-reaching afflictions of stressful work to workers' health. Therefore, joint efforts are required from stakeholders, professionals and national/international organizations to improve healthy work and, by doing so, to reduce the burden of work-stress related disease.

NOTE

1. Acknowledgement: Some paragraphs of this chapter are modified from the review chapter Siegrist, J. (2009). Job control and reward: effects on well being. In S. Cartwright and C.C. Cooper (Eds.), *The Oxford handbook of organizational well-being* (pp. 109–132). Oxford, UK: Oxford University Press.

REFERENCES

Ala-Mursula, L., Vahtera, J., Linna, A., Pentti, J., & Kivimäki, M. (2005). Employee worktime control moderates the effects of job strain and effort-reward imbalance on sickness absence: the 10-Town Study. *Journal of Epidemiology and Community Health, 59,* 851–857.

Aust, B., Peter, R., & Siegrist, J. (1997). Stress management in bus drivers: a pilot study based on the model of effort-reward imbalance. *International Journal of Stress Management, 4,* 297–305.

Bellingrath, S., Rohfelder, N., & Kudielka, B. M. (2010). Healthy working scholl teachers with high effort-reward-imbalance and overcommitment show increased pro-inflammatory immune activity and a dampeened innate immune defence. *Brain, Behaviour and Immunology, 24,* 1332–1339.

Bellingrath, S., Weigl, T., & Kudielka, B.M. (2008). Cortisol dysregulation in school teachers in relation to burnout, vital exhaustion, and effort-reward imbalance. *Biological Psychology 78,* 104–113.

Biron, C., Cooper, C.L., & Bond, F.W. (2009). Mediators and moderators of organizational inerventions to prevent occupational stress. In S. Cartwright & C.L. Cooper (Eds.), *The Oxford handbook of organizational well-being* (pp. 441–465). Oxford, UK: Oxford University Press.

Black, C. (2008). *Working for a healthier tomorrow.* London, UK: TSO.

Bosma, H., Peter, R., Siegrist, J., & Marmot, M. (1998). Two alternative job stress models and the risk of coronary heart disease. *American Journal of Public Health 88,* 68–74.

Bourbonnais, R., Brisson, C., Vinet, A., Vezina, M., & Lower, A. (2006). Development and implementation of a participative intervention to improve the psychosocial work environment and mental health in an acute care hospital. *Occupational and Environmental Medicine, 63,* 326–334.

Bourbonnais, R., Brisson, C., & Vezina, M. (2011). Long-term effects of an intervention on psychosocial work factors among healthcare professionals in a hospital setting. *Occupational & Environmental Medicine, 68,* 479–486.

Chandola, T., Marmot, M., & Siegrist, J. (2007). Failed reciprocity in close social relationships and health: Findings from the Whitehall II study. *Journal of Psychosomatic Research, 63,* 403–411.

de Jonge, J., van der Linden, S., Schaufeli, W., Peter, R., & Siegrist, J. (2008). Factorial invariance and stability of the Effort-Reward Imbalance Scales: a longitudinal analysis of two samples with different time lags. *International Journal of Behavioural Medicine, 15*(1), 62–72.

Dragano, N., Siegrist, J., & Wahrendorf, M. (2011). Welfare regimes, labour policies and unhealthy psychosocial working conditions: A comparative study with 9917 older employees from 12 European countries. *Journal of Epidemiology and Community Health, 65,* 793–799.

Eller, N. H., Netterstrøm, B., Gyntelberg, F., Kristensen, T. S., Nielsen, F., Steptoe, A., & Theorell, T. (2009). Work-related psychosocial factors and the development of ischemic heart disease. *Cardiology Review, 17,* 83–97.

Griep, R.H., Rotenberg, L., Vasconcellos, A.G., Landsbergis, P., Comaru, C. M., & Alves, M. G. (2009). The psychometric properties of demand-control and effort-reward imbalance scales among Brazilian nurses. *International Archives of Occupational and Environmental, 82*(10), 1163–1172.

Hamer, M., Williams, E., Vuonovirta, R., Giacobazzi, P., Gibson, E.L., & Steptoe, A. (2006). The effects of effort-reward imbalance on inflammatory and cardiovascular responses to mental stress. *Psychosomatic Medicine, 68,* 408–413.

Head, J., Kivimäki, M., Siegrist, J., Ferrie, J., Vahtera, J., Shipley, M. J., & Marmot, M. (2007) Effort-reward imbalance and relational injustice at work predict sickness absence: the Whitehall II study. *Journal of Psychosomatic Research 63*, 433–440.

Henry, J.P., & Stephens, P.M. (1977). *Stress, health, and the social environment.* New York, NY: Springer.

Hurwitz Eller, N., Netterstrom, B., & Hansen, A.M. (2006). Psychosocial factors at home and at work and levels of salivary cortisol. *Biological Psychology, 7*, 280–287.

Johnson, J.V., & Hall, E.M. (1988). Job strain, workplace social support and cardiovascular disease: A cross sectional study of a random sample of the Swedish working population. *American Journal of Public Health, 78*, 1336–1342.

Johnston, D.W., Beedie, A., & Jones, M.C. (2006). Using computerized ambulatory diaries for the assessment of job characteristics and work-related stress in nurses. *Work & Stress, 20*(2), 163–172.

Karasek, R.A., & Theorell, T. (1990). *Healthy work.* New York, NY: Basic Books.

Karasek, R., Brisson, C., Kawakami, N. Houtman, I., Bongers, P., & Amick, B. (1998). The job content questionnaire (JCQ): an instrument for internationally comparative assessment of psychosocial job characteristics. *Journal of Occupational Health Psychology, 3*, 322–355.

Kelloway, E.K., & Barling, J. (2010). Leadership development as an intervention in occupational health psychology. *Work & Stress 24*, 260–279

Kivimäki, M., Leino-Arjas, P., Luukonen, R., Riihimäki, H., Vahtera, J., & Kirjonen, J. (2002). Work stress and risk of cardiovascular mortality: Prospective cohort study of industrial employees. *British Medical Journal, 325*, 857–861.

Kivimäki, M., Virtanen, M., Elovainio, M., Kouvonen, A., Väänänen, A., & Vahtera, J. (2006). Work stress in the etiology of coronary heart disease—A meta-analysis. *Scandinavian Journal of Work, Environment and Health, 32*, 431–442.

Krause, N., Brand, R. J., Kauhanen, J., Kaplan, G. A., Syme, S. L., Wong, C. C., & Salonen, J. T. (2009). Work time an 11-year progression of carotid atherosclerosis in middle-aged Finnish men. *Preventing Chronic Disease, 6*, 1–20.

Kuper, H., Singh-Manoux, A., Siegrist, J., & Marmot, M. (2002). When reciprocity fails: effort-reward imbalance in relation to coronary heart disease and health functioning within the Whitehall II Study. *Occupational and Environmental Medicine, 59*, 777–784.

Landsbergis, P.A. (2003). The changing organization of work and the safety and health of working people: a commentary. *Journal of Occupational and Environmental Medicine, 11*, 61–71.

Landsbergis, P.A. (2009). Interventions to reduce job stress and improve work organization and worker health. In P.L. Schnall, M. Dobson, & E. Rosskam (Eds.), *Unhealthy work* (pp. 193–209). Amityville, NY: Baywood Publishing Company.

Leineweber, C., Wege, N., Westerlund, H., Theorell, T., Wahrendorf, M., & Siegrist, J. (2010). How valid is a short measure of effort-reward imbalance at work? A replication study from Sweden. *Occupational and Environmental Medicine, 67*, 526–531.

Li, J., Shang, L., Wang, T., & Siegrist, J. (2010). Measuring effort-reward imbalance in school settings: A novel approach and its association with self-rated health. *Journal of Epidemiology / Japan Epidemiological Association 20*, 111–118.

Limm, H., Gündel, H., Heinmüller, M., Marten-Mittag, B., Nater, U. M., Siegrist, J., & Angerer, P. (2011). Stress management interventions in the workplace improve stress rectivity: A randomised controlled trial. *Occupational & Environmental Medicine, 68,* 126–133.

Lynch, J., Krause, N., Kaplan, G.A., Tuomilehto, J., & Salonen, J.T. (1997). Work place conditions, socioeconomic status, and the risk of mortality and acute myocardial infarction: the Kuopio ischemic heart disease risk factor study. *American Journal of Public Health, 87,* 617–622.

Mathers, C.D., Lopez, A.D., & Murray, C.J.L. (2006). The burden of disease and mortality by condition: data, methods, and results for 2001. In A.D. Lopez, C.D. Mathers, M. Ezzati et al. (Eds.), *Global burden of disease and risk factors,* 45–234.

McEwen, B. (1998). Protective and damaging effects of stress mediators. *New England Journal of Medicine, 338,* 171–179.

Ostry, A.S., & Spiegel, J.M. (2004). Labor markets and employment insecurity: impacts of globalization on the healthcare workforce. *International Journal of Occupational and Environmental Health, 10,* 368–374.

Rau, R., Morling, K., & Rösler, U. (2010). Is there a relationship between major depression and both objectively assessed and perceived demands and control? *Work & Stress, 24,* 88–106.

Schnall, P.L., Dobson, M., & Rosskam, E. (Eds). (2009). *Unhealthy work: Causes, consequences and cures.* Amityville, NY: Baywood Press.

Schultz, W., Dayan, P., Montague, P.R. (1997). A neural substrate of prediction and reward. *Science 275,* 1593–1599.

Siegrist, J. (1996). Adverse health effects of high-effort/low-reward conditions. Journal of Occupational Health Psychology, 1, 27–41.

Siegrist, J. (2009). Unfair exchange and health: Social bases of stress-related diseases. *Social Theory and Health,* 7(4), 305–317.

Siegrist, J., & Dragano, N. (2008). Psychosocial stress and disease risks in occupational life. Results of international studies on the demand-control and the effort-reward imbalance models. *Bundesgesundheitsblatt–Gesundheitsforschung Gesundheitsschutz, 51,* 305–312.

Siegrist, J., Peter, R., Junge, A., Cremer, P., & Seidel, D. (1990). Low status control, high effort at work and ischemic heart disease: Prospective evidence from blue-collar men. *Social Science & Medicine, 31,* 1127–1134.

Siegrist, J., & Rödel, A. (2006). Work stress and health risk behaviour. *Scandinavian Journal of Work and Environmental Health, 32,* 473–481.

Siegrist, J., Starke, D., Chandola, T. et al. (2004). The measurement of Effort-Reward Imbalance at work: European comparisons. *Social Science & Medicine, 58*(8), 1483–1499.

Siegrist, J., Wege, N., Pühlhofer, F., & Wahredorf, M. (2009) A short generic measure of work stress in the era of globailzation: effort reward imbalance. *International Archives of Occupational and Environmental Health, 82,* 1005–1013.

Stansfeld, S.A., & Marmot, M. (Eds.). (2002), *Stress and the heart.* London, UK: BMJ Publishing.

Steptoe, A., Siegrist, J., Kirschbaum, C., & Marmot, M. (2004). Effort–reward imbalance, overcommitment, and measures of cortisol and blood pressure over the working day. *Psychosomatic Medicine, 66,* 323-329.

Tsutsumi, A., & Kawakami, A. (2004). A review of empirical studies on the model of effort–reward imbalance at work: Reducing occupational stress by implementing a new theory. Social Science & Medicine, 59, 2335–2359.

Tsutsumi, A., Nagami, M., Morimoto, K., & Matoba, T. (2002). Responsiveness of measures in the effort–reward imbalance questionnaire to organisational change: A validation study. *Journal of Psychosomatic, 52,* 249–256.

van Vegchel, N., de Jonge, J., Bosma, H., & Schaufeli, W. (2005). Reviewing the effort–reward imbalance model: drawing up the balance of 45 empirical studies. *Social Science & Medicine, 60,* 1117–1131.

Vrijkotte, D.G.M., Doornen, L.J.P van, & de Geus, E.J.C. (2000). Effect of work stress on ambulatory blood pressure, heart rate, and heart rate variability. *Hypertension 35,* 880–86.

Wahrendorf, M., Ribet, C., Zins, M., Goldberg, M., & Siegrist, J. (2010). Perceived reciprocity in social exchange and health functioning in early old age: Prospective findings from the GAZEL study. *Aging & Mental Health, 14,* 425–432.

Weiner, H. (1992). *Perturbing the organism. The biology of stressful experience.* Chicago, IL: Chicago University Press.

Wirtz, P.H., Siegrist, J., Rimmele, U., & Ehlert, U. (2008). Higher overcommitment to work is associated with lower norepinephrine secretion before and after acute psychosocial stress in men. *Psychoneuroendocrinology, 33,* 92–99.

CHAPTER 6

THAT WASN'T TOO STRESSFUL, OR WAS IT

Physiological Stress Responses to Regulatory Focus (Mis)Match

Chad Ian Peddie, Julie A. Agar,
Kate A. LaPort, and Lois E. Tetrick
George Mason University

ABSTRACT

There has been a widespread call for researchers and practitioners to develop more integrated and comprehensive approaches to health promotion in the workplace. Regulatory focus theory may provide a key, unexplored ingredient to understanding the physiological impact of work tasks. Previous research suggests that when individuals with a chronic (or trait-like) regulatory focus operate under conditions that induce a (state-like) focus that does not coincide with the chronic focus, they tend to "feel less right" and find tasks less pleasant and more stressful (Cesario & Higgins, 2008). The current study examined the direct link between regulatory focus (mis)match and both self-reported and physiological measures of stress in a laboratory setting. Participants' state regulatory focus was manipulated while completing a typing task.

Coping and Prevention, pages 93–108

> Results revealed significant differences in systolic blood pressure measurement based on match and mismatch conditions, with those in a regulatory focus mismatch exhibiting increasing systolic blood pressure.

There has been a widespread call for researchers and practitioners to develop more integrated and comprehensive approaches to health promotion in the workplace (Aust & Ducki, 2004; Polanyi, Frank, Shannon, Sullivan, & Lavis, 2000; Syme, 1996). Some initiatives have focused on inducing positive change in employees' behavior by increasing physical activity in the workplace (Dugdill & Coffey, 2009; Tavares & Plotnikoff, 2008) or providing smoking cessation programs (Bergstrom et al., 2008; Eriksen & Gottlieb, 1998; O'Donnell, 2006). Other research has examined the impact that characteristics of the job itself may have on employee health, well-being, performance, absenteeism, and healthcare costs (Ganster, Fox, & Dwyer, 2001; Wellens, & Smith, 2006; Westerlund, Theorell, & Alfredsson, 2004).

While job characteristics such as overtime requirements, autonomy, job barriers, and time pressure have been explored extensively, the current chapter looks to regulatory focus theory (Higgins, 1997, 1998) to provide additional insight into employee well-being and occupational stress research. Regulatory focus theory posits that individuals possess chronic preferences for goal attainment strategies. When there is a match between an individual's chronic preference and the requirements of a specific situation (e.g., framing of the job task), research has demonstrated a positive impact on that individual's motivation (Spiegel, Grant-Pillow, & Higgins, 2004), task performance (Keller & Bless, 2006), and confidence regarding decision-making (Higgins, 2000).

Drawing from the person–environment fit and stress literature, as well as previous research tying regulatory focus mismatch to "feeling less right" about a task or activity (Cesario & Higgins, 2008) and finding a task less pleasant and more stressful (Latimer et al., 2008), the current chapter details a study that explores the hypothesis that being in a regulatory focus match, wherein a person's chronic regulatory focus and the state regulatory focus correspond to each other, results in lower levels of stress. Results from this study reflect the impact of occupational task instructions, which either (1) match an individual's chronic regulatory focus or (2) mismatch an individual's chronic regulatory focus, on an individual's self-reported stress levels, ambulatory blood pressure, and performance.

This study was designed to investigate whether there is a relationship between regulatory focus match and occupational stress. To do so, we begin by presenting an overview of regulatory focus theory and the concept of regulatory focus (mis)match. We then provide background information, including health outcome data, to explain why understanding physiological stress responses is important to employee well-being and performance.

After presenting the study's methodology and findings, we conclude with a discussion of the implications the results hold for regulatory focus theory, occupational health psychology, and future research.

REGULATORY FOCUS THEORY

Regulatory focus theory is a motivational theory whose foundation can be attributed to the work of Higgins and his colleagues who argue that individuals have a stable orientation that results in them preferring particular regulatory strategies when pursuing goals (Higgins, 1997, 1998). Higgins (1997, 1998) specifically identifies two types of goal-striving orientations: promotion and prevention (Higgins, 1997, 1998). Promotion strategies revolve around advancement, achievement, accomplishments, and gains for the individual (Higgins, 1996). The driver of behavior, with regard to this focus, is a need for development and growth captured by setting ideal and hoped-for goals (Carver & Scheier, 1998). People with a promotion focus are therefore concerned with establishing the presence of outcomes associated with success (Higgins & Tykocinski, 1992). These individuals are characterized by their *eagerness* to reach the desired end-state of accomplishment (Crowe & Higgins, 1997).

Prevention strategies, on the other hand, focus on obligations, safety, and responsibilities (Higgins, 1996). Individuals with a prevention focus are therefore concerned with avoiding the presence of outcomes associated with failure. This focus is driven by a need for protection from harm to self, which manifests through setting *feared* and *ought* goals (Carver & Scheier, 1998). These goals are set to represent the duties that one is obligated to perform. People with a prevention focus are characterized by *vigilance* as a means to ensure safety and protect against losses.

It is important to note that Higgins and colleagues view regulatory focus both as a relatively stable chronic disposition and as a psychological state that can be primed by the situation. Individual differences in the extent to which a person is promotion or prevention focused are referred to as an individuals' "chronic regulatory focus." In short, those individuals with a chronic promotion focus tend to actively seek outcomes associated with success, are more open to change, and look toward the future, valuing achievement and advancement. On the other hand, individuals with a chronic prevention focus wish to avoid outcomes associated with failure, prefer stability, and work to fulfill responsibilities and obligations (Higgins 1997, 1998). In contrast to this chronic regulatory focus, promotion and prevention foci can also be temporarily induced or primed by situational variables such as task requirements. This is referred to as "state regulatory focus."

REGULATORY FOCUS MATCH

When individuals' chronic tendencies correspond to their state regulatory focus, they are said to be in a regulatory focus match (Higgins, 2000). Previous research has demonstrated a number of positive effects related to individuals working under conditions that match their chronic regulatory focus. For example, individuals in a regulatory focus match have been found to be more motivated (Spiegel et al., 2004) and to perform better (Keller & Bless, 2006). Other research has found that being in a regulatory focus match leads to individuals feeling better about a situation or decision (Cesario & Higgins, 2008; Larkin, Pines, & LaPort, 2007). For example, Cesario and Higgins (2008) asked college students to watch a video in which information was either presented in an eager (promotion) delivery style or a vigilant (prevention) delivery style. Participants in a regulatory focus match reported "feeling right" about the content of the video significantly more than those in a regulatory focus mismatch.

Another study suggests that a regulatory focus match predicts positive feelings, such as rating an activity as pleasant, enjoyable, and relaxing, as opposed to stressful (Latimer et al., 2008). It is important to remember that since regulatory focus match results in positive outcomes and emotions, regulatory focus mismatch appears to have the opposite influence—including not "feeling as right" and finding an activity to be less pleasant, not as enjoyable, and more stressful (Cesario & Higgins, 2008; Latimer et al., 2008).

What is the explanation for this? Higgins (1997) explains regulatory focus match as reducing the discrepancy between one's desired end-state and the way in which that end-state is approached. This is reminiscent of theories of person–environment fit. In this stream of research, individuals have been shown to experience more positive work-related outcomes when they are in work environments that are congruent with their personal values, skills, knowledge, abilities, and needs (Kristof-Brown, Zimmerman, & Johnson, 2005; Spokane, Meir, & Catalano, 2000; Tinsley, 2000). Conversely, individuals who do not fit with their environments experience less job satisfaction, less organizational commitment, lower organizational identity (Edwards & Cable, 2009), and particularly pertinent to the present study, greater stress symptoms (Pithers & Soden, 1999; Saks & Ashforth, 1997). Mapped onto the regulatory focus theory framework, negative results would be expected when there is a discrepancy between a person's characteristics (i.e., chronic regulatory focus tendencies) and their environment (i.e., situationally determined regulatory focus) (Edwards & Cooper, 1990; Saks & Ashforth, 1997). Consistent with the person–environment fit literature, we hypothesize the following:

Hypothesis 1a: *Individuals in a regulatory focus mismatch report significantly higher levels of stress than those working in a regulatory focus match.*

PHYSIOLOGICAL STRESS RESPONSES

Corresponding with this hypothesis, since we expect participants to report higher levels of stress in a regulatory focus mismatch, we should also expect to see similar results if we observe actual physiological indicators of stress. Measuring elevations in blood pressure is one strategy we can use to gauge cardiovascular reactivity to stress. Cardiovascular reactivity can be conceptualized as a change in value from some baseline measure to values rendered during a stressful event (Kelsey, Ornduff, & Alpert, 2007). The current study focuses on elevations in blood pressure as a key form of cardiovascular reactivity. In order to fully understand our additional hypotheses, it is important to know that blood pressure consists of two forces. One of these types of pressure, the systolic pressure, is generated by the heart pumping blood into the arteries. The other type of pressure, the diastolic pressure, is the pressure in vessels between heart beats (American Heart Association, 2008).

In addition to investigating whether regulatory focus mismatch is related to self-reported stress, the study reported here directly examines the link between regulatory focus match and physiological indicators of stress, specifically elevations in blood pressure. Therefore, we propose the following hypotheses:

Hypothesis 1b: *Individuals with a regulatory focus mismatch experience significantly higher systolic blood pressure changes than those working in a regulatory focus match.*

Hypothesis 1c: *Individuals in a regulatory focus mismatch experience significantly higher diastolic blood pressure changes than those working in a regulatory focus match.*

METHOD

To experimentally examine these hypotheses, data were collected from undergraduate students (11 men and 50 women) from a medium-sized university in the Mid-Atlantic region of the United States. The average age of participants was 20.5 years and they identified themselves as 44% Caucasian, 15% Asian, 13% African American, 13% Hispanic, and 15% as other. When these participants arrived at the lab they were asked to complete the measure of chronic regulatory focus (Lockwood, Jordan, & Kunda, 2002) and were then randomly assigned to one of two conditions. Their assigned condition determined their performance strategy for both a distracter task and the main performance task. The two conditions were:

1. Eagerness: Participants were asked to perform tasks as *quickly* as possible, where the amount completed was more important than the accuracy. These instructions primed participants to pursue a promotion goal attainment strategy and were similar to those used in Spiegel et al. (2004).
2. Vigilance: Participants were asked to perform tasks as *accurately* as possible, where the precision of responses was more important than the amount completed. These instructions primed a prevention strategy for participants and were similar to the instructions used in previous regulatory focus research (Spiegel et al., 2004).

After selection of condition the dominant arm of participants was fitted with an ambulatory blood pressure monitor, which took readings at five-minute intervals throughout the study session. The first activity participants completed was a computer-administered distracter task involving completion of a number of math problems for ten minutes. The math problems were the same for both conditions; however, depending on the assigned condition, participants were requested to complete the task either as accurately (prevention-focused condition) or quickly (promotion-focused condition) as possible.

Following completion of the distracter task was a computer-administered typing exercise. Participants were directed to type for twenty minutes using their non-dominant hand. According to their assigned condition, they were told that *speed* (typing as much as you can in an allotted time—promotion-focused condition) or *accuracy* (limiting errors—prevention-focused condition) was important. These instructions were similar in nature to those used by Spiegel et al. (2004), in which a promotion focus was induced by asking participants to capture as many details as possible and a prevention focus was induced by asking them to not forget any details. Finally, participants were asked to fill out the Dundee Stress State Questionnaire to determine their self-reported stress levels.

MEASURES

Performance

The typing task was conducted with *Stamina Typing Tutor.* This program presents participants with text that is required to be typed. This program automatically records measures of both speed (CPM) and accuracy (error), which is represented by the total number of keystrokes made by a participant that do not correspond to the displayed character. The program allows for customized trail time spans; in other words, it is possible to set a specific amount of time between the start of a typing trail until the point when results are displayed. It was decided that two measurements of participant performance would be collected. The first measure was taken halfway through the task (10 minutes) and a second measure at the end of the task (20 minutes).

Physiological Stress Response

Participants' physiological stress reactions were measured by taking their blood pressure with the Tiba Medical SE-25S Ambulatory Blood Pressure Monitor at five-minute intervals throughout the performance task. A baseline measure of blood pressure was recorded immediately prior to the performance task while participants completed the math task.

Self-reported Stress

Self-reported stress of participants was assessed via the Dundee Stress State Questionnaire (Matthews, Joyner, Gilliland, Campbell, Huggins, & Falconer, 1999). The 96-item measure was designed to assess transient states rather than traits and can be broken down into three higher-order stress dimensions: task engagement, distress, and worry (Matthews et al., 2002). Sample items include "Please rate your FRUSTRATION: How discouraged, irritated, stressed and annoyed did you feel during the task?" and "Please rate the TEMPORAL DEMAND of the task: How much time pressure did you feel due to the pace at which the task elements occurred?"

Chronic Regulatory Focus

Participants completed Lockwood et al.'s (2002) measure of school-based chronic regulatory focus. This 18-item self-report measure was chosen because of the appropriateness of the school context for our undergraduate participant population (Schmit, Ryan, Stierwalt, & Powell, 1995). Sample items include "My major goal in school right now is to achieve my academic ambitions" and "My major goal in school right now is to avoid becoming an academic failure." Participants were asked to respond to these statements on a scale from 1 (not at all true of me) to 9 (very true of me). Each participant received scores on the nine-item promotion ($\alpha = .86$) and nine-item prevention ($\alpha = .91$) subscales. For the purposes of this study, individuals were identified as either prevention- or promotion-focused based on a median split of their promotion and prevention scores following the strategy used by Cesario, Grant, and Higgins (2004). Thus each participant had a single categorical chronic regulatory focus score (0 = Prevention, 1 = Promotion).

(Mis)Match

A categorical variable was computed based on congruence between assigned condition and chronic regulatory focus to indicate whether each participant was in the match or mismatch condition (0 = mismatch, 1 = match). For example, if a participant was categorized as having a chronic promotion focus and they received speed task instructions, they were categorized as having a "match" between their chronic and state regulatory focus. The percentage of participants in the match category (44%) was relatively equal to the percentage of participants in the mismatch category (53%).

RESULTS

Stress

Self-Reported Stress

This study hypothesized that participants in a match condition would report significantly less stress than those in a mismatch condition (Hypothesis 1a). Contrary to expectations, an independent samples t-test revealed that participants in a match versus mismatch condition did not differ significantly in self-reported stress. None of the three Dundee Stress State Questionnaire subscales (worried, engaged, or distressed) showed a statistically significant difference between those in the match condition and those in the mismatch condition.

Physiological Stress

Means and standard deviations of the major variables of interest can be seen in Table 6.1. To specifically test Hypotheses 1b and 1c, the impact of regulatory focus match on systolic and diastolic blood pressure readings was examined using two repeated measures Analyses of Covariance. We examined blood pressure measurements for the first, second, third, and fourth intervals, which were collected five, ten, fifteen, and twenty minutes after the commencement of the performance task. To account for initial differences on the between-subjects variable, the participants' baseline sys-

TABLE 6.1 Means and Standard Deviations of Systolic and Diastolic Blood Pressure Across Time by (Mis)match

	Measurement Interval			
	1	2	3	4
Match				
Systolic	112.56 (15.98)	113.79 (19.68)	111.29 (16.19)	110.67 (17.80)
Diastolic	69.03 (10.27)	66.03 (11.94)	65.94 (9.45)	64.77 (9.47)
Mismatch				
Systolic	111.29 (11.68)	112.10 (15.27)	113.90 (18.92)	119.75 (24.16)
Diastolic	67.43 (8.36)	68.74 (13.35)	69.34 (13.01)	70.57 (13.68)
Total				
Systolic	112.19 (13.76)	114.31 (19.05)	113.04 (17.57)	115.65 (21.39)
Diastolic	67.94 (9.41)	68.10 (14.01)	67.51 (11.61)	67.71 (12.10)

Note: Measurement Interval 1 corresponds to blood pressure five minutes after commencement of the task; Measurement Interval 2 corresponds to blood pressure ten minutes after commencement of the task; Measurement Interval 3 corresponds to blood pressure fifteen minutes after commencement of the task; Measurement Interval 4 corresponds to blood pressure twenty minutes after commencement of the task.

tolic and diastolic blood pressure measurements were used as covariates (Llabre, Spitzer, Saab, Ironson, & Schneiderman, 1991).

With regards to systolic blood pressure readings, a significant interaction between (mis)match and systolic blood pressure measurements was found. A plot of this interaction (Figure 6.1) reveals increasing systolic blood pressure for those in the mismatch condition, thus supporting our second hypothesis. A second repeated measures analysis of covariance examining diastolic blood pressure revealed no significant interaction between (mis) match and diastolic blood pressure measurements, although an examination of the graph (Figure 6.2) reveals a trend in the hypothesized direction.

DISCUSSION

The above results reveal interesting outcomes associated with the performance of tasks in both cases of regulatory match and mismatch. Support was not found for the hypothesis that individuals with a regulatory focus mismatch would report higher levels of stress. In contrast to the self-reported stress results, however, the study reported here did find support for the hypothesis that individuals with a regulatory focus mismatch would experience significantly higher systolic blood pressure changes than those individuals in a regulatory focus match. Statistically significant results were not found for diastolic blood pressure changes, but an examination of both

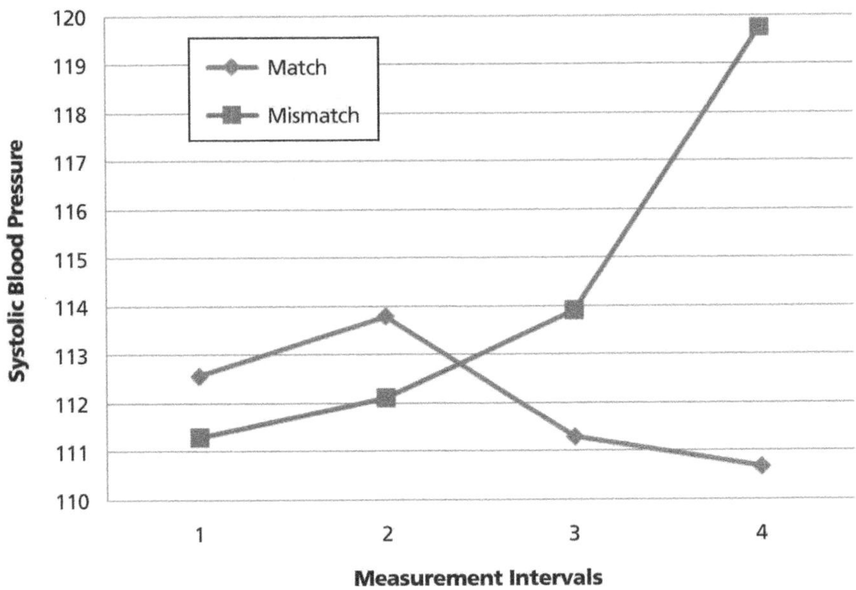

Figure 6.1 Regulatory focus mis(match) systolic blood pressure over time. Measurement Interval 1 corresponds to blood pressure five minutes after commencement of the task; Measurement Interval 2 corresponds to blood pressure ten minutes after commencement of the task; Measurement Interval 3 corresponds to blood pressure fifteen minutes after commencement of the task; Measurement Interval 4 corresponds to blood pressure twenty minutes after commencement of the task.

plots (see Figures 6.1 and 6.2) revealed similar trends for both the diastolic and systolic blood pressure measurements at the four intervals measured.

In further consideration of the nature of diastolic blood pressure, a significant effect of regulatory focus mismatch on elevations in systolic blood pressure, but not diastolic, should not be alarming. It has been established that when considering cardiovascular reactivity to effort, systolic blood pressure is predictably influenced by the contractility of heart muscle tissues and is thus considered a reliable index of effort (Wright, 1996). In fact, of cardiovascular parameters (i.e., systolic blood pressure, diastolic blood pressure, and pulse), systolic blood pressure has been conceptualized as the most sensitive response to experienced difficulty when engaged in a task (de Burgo & Gendolla, 2009). This sensitivity is thought to be due to the relationship between systolic blood pressure and the sympathetic nervous system. This system is responsible for regulating behavior in reaction to stress stimuli and thus registering the physiological effects of stress reactions (Sherman, Bunyan, Creswell, & Jaremka, 2009). The similar pattern displayed by diastolic blood pressure (approaching, although not statisti-

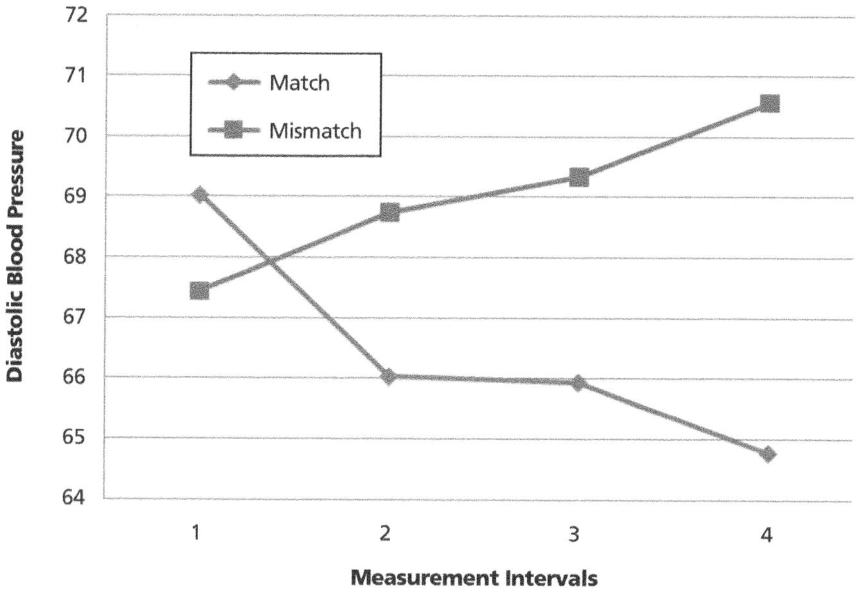

Figure 6.2 Regulatory focus mis(match) systolic blood pressure over time. Measurement Interval 1 corresponds to blood pressure five minutes after commencement of the task; Measurement Interval 2 corresponds to blood pressure ten minutes after commencement of the task; Measurement Interval 3 corresponds to blood pressure fifteen minutes after commencement of the task; Measurement Interval 4 corresponds to blood pressure twenty minutes after commencement of the task.

cally significant) is consistent with previous research demonstrating that when individuals experience task-related difficulty, cardiovascular response can be high enough that it increases the pressure within blood vessels between heart beats (i.e., diastolic pressure), but to a considerably lesser degree than on systolic pressure.

The findings of the current study have important implications for how we study stress in organizational settings. Historically, physiological measures of stress, such as blood pressure, have been heavily relied upon in the health psychology stress literature, but less so by industrial-organizational psychologists. The incorporation of physiological measures of stress reactions may contribute to our understanding of stress responses, perhaps in a more reliable and unbiased nature, than traditional self-reports. Additionally, physiological measures may prove more effective in potentially measuring more situation-specific aspects of stress reactions than the more chronic-natured self-reports. The failure of the self-report measure of stress to show differences among groups in the context of the regulatory focus mismatch demonstrates that, as others have posited in the past (Schwartz,

Pickering, & Landsbergis, 1996), employees may not always be aware of their manifestations of physiological stress until it has persisted for some period of time or the cumulative effect has begun to take a toll on their health. To our knowledge, there has been no empirical research investigating this line of thought, making it an important area worthy of investigation in future research.

The study's findings also have implications for employee well-being. A paradigm shift in the medical literature has resulted in systolic blood pressure being identified as the most accurate and primary criterion for gauging hypertension in certain populations. Hypertension due to elevations of systolic blood pressure has been associated with stroke, myocardial infarction, heart failure, kidney failure, and overall cardiovascular disease morbidity and mortality (Izzo, Levy, & Black, 2000). Cardiovascular disease, in particular, has been the leading cause of death in the United States for the past 80 years, with 652,091 Americans succumbing to heart disease and related complications each year (American Heart Association, 2008). Therefore, our finding that systolic blood pressure was significantly elevated under conditions of regulatory focus mismatch have particularly important implications for employee health outcomes.

Considering that occupational stress costs U.S. businesses roughly $300 billion per year as a result of absenteeism, turnover, lowered productivity, and medical, legal, and insurance fees (American Psychological Association, 2007), strategies for reducing stress on the job could have major implications for a company's bottom line. There are several ways that the results of this study could be generalized to a work setting in order to reduce job stress. One strategy might be to frame job tasks in such a way that they match an employee's regulatory focus. For example, if a manager were asking an employee with a prevention focus to complete a task, he or she might want to focus on the importance of not making mistakes or paying very close attention to detail. Another strategy might be more selection oriented. Although a selection strategy might not be applicable for the majority of jobs today, it could still be relevant for certain industries, such as manufacturing, where a factory line worker who makes minimal mistakes would be highly valued. Obviously, these are just starting points, and further research is needed outside of the laboratory before these strategies can actually be utilized.

Another aspect of this study that holds implications for organizations concerns the impact of regulatory focus match and mismatch on performance results. Although this study did not specifically hypothesize an effect on task performance levels, it is important to realize that subsequent analyses of performance data obtained in this study found that individuals in both match and mismatch conditions performed similarly. It is reassuring to consider that potentially reframing tasks to match the focus of an individual worker may result in reduced stress-related health outcomes with no sacrifice to performance levels. As illustrated above, the costs to organizations in retroactively dealing with occupational stressors are staggering. The results from the current study show that these very organizations might realize bottom-line benefits by proactively and strategically designing approaches to task completion to individual employees.

Additionally, consideration of these performance data stand in contradiction to some previous research demonstrating superior levels of performance when regulatory focus of individuals matched task procedures (e.g., Keller & Bless, 2006; Shah, Higgins, & Friedman, 1998). A potential explanation of these inconsistencies might lie in the nature of the tasks employed in the various studies. Previous research looked at the impact of regulatory focus match on two types of tasks that shared a central feature: cognitive flexibility. While arguably Keller and Bless' (2006) assessment of participant ability to generate methods of persevering with a new lifestyle (e.g., life after a leg amputation) reflects an exercise in thinking flexibly to adapt to change, Shah and colleagues' (1998) focus on anagram solving skills relates directly to cognitive flexibility (Ghacibeh, Shenker, Shenal, Uthman, & Heilman, 2006). Only assessing the impact of regulatory match/mismatch on tasks focusing on cognitive flexibility leaves a breadth of tasks in which the performance/regulatory focus match relationship may vary. When tasks tend to be more straightforward, such as in the present typing task where the demands of performance are more restrictive, the performance variability may be less sensitive to regulatory focus match.

Several limitations of this study need to be acknowledged. First, the study was conducted in a laboratory with student participants, which raises the question of whether these findings can be generalized to employees in a work setting. However, by randomly assigning participants to experimental conditions, we were able to control for extraneous variables that might have otherwise influenced our findings. A second limitation was that the time spent tracking the blood pressure of each participant was relatively short, therefore not allowing for long-term assessment of physiological stress responses. Although short-lived, the effects of regulatory focus (mis)match were seen throughout the course of the experiment, which included multiple measures of systolic and diastolic blood pressure.

The limited understanding of the impact on individuals of a specific chronic regulatory focus strategy working under situations requiring the alternative foci rests on a relatively small body of literature. The findings gleaned from the current study add to knowledge within this field. To date, this is the pioneer inspection of stress responses to regulatory focus (mis) match. Although more research investigating the effects of regulatory focus (mis)match is needed to fully understand whether findings from the current study translate to working professional populations over greater durations of task engagement, the findings reported here lay a blueprint of what outcomes additional samples should consider.

REFERENCES

American Heart Association. (2008). *Heart disease and stroke statistics—2009 update.* Dallas, TX: Statistics Committee and Stroke Statistics Subcommittee.

American Psychological Association. (2007, August 22). *Don't let workplace stress ruin your Labor day holiday.* Retrieved from http://www.apa.org/news/press /releases/2007/08/workplace-stress.aspx

Aust, B., & Ducki, A. (2004). Comprehensive health interventions at the workplace: Experiences with health circles in Germany. *Journal of Occupational Health Psychology, 9*,258–270.

Bergstrom, G., Bjorklunda, C., Fried, I., Lisspers, J., Nathell, L., Hermansson, U.,...Jensen, I. B. (2008). A comprehensive workplace intervention and its outcome with regards to lifestyle, health, and sick leave: The AHA study. *Work: Journal of Prevention, Assessment, and Rehabilitation, 31,* 167–180.

Carver, C. S., & Scheier, M. F. (1998). *On the self-regulation of behavior.* New York, NY: Cambridge University Press

Cesario, J., Grant, H., & Higgins, E. T. (2004). Regulatory fit and persuasion: Transfer from 'feeling right.' *Journal of Personality and Social Psychology, 86,* 388–404.

Cesario, J., & Higgins, E. T. (2008). Making message recipients 'feel right': How nonverbal cues can increase persuasion. *Psychological Science, 19,* 415–420.

Crowe, E., & Higgins, E. T. (1997). Regulatory focus and strategic inclinations: Promotion and prevention in decision-making. *Organizational Behavior and Human Decision Processes, 69,* 117–132.

de Burgo, J., & Gendolla, G. H. E. (2009). Are moods motivational states? A study on effort-related cardiovascular response. *Emotion. 9,* 892–897.

Dugdill, L., & Coffey, M. (2009). Developing physically active workplaces. In L. Dugdill, D. Crone, & R. Murphy (Eds.), *Physical activity and health promotion: Evidence-based approaches to practice* (pp. 130–149). Hoboken, NJ: Wiley-Blackwell.

Edwards, J. R., & Cable, D. M. (2009). The value of value congruence. *Journal of Applied Psychology, 94,* 654–677.

Edwards, J. R., & Cooper, C. L. (1990). The person–environment fit approach to stress: Recurring problems and some suggested solutions. *Journal of Organizational Behavior, 11,* 293–307.

Eriksen, M. P., Gottlieb, N. H. (1998). A review of the health impact of smoking control at the workplace. *American Journal of Health Promotion, 13,* 83–104.

Ganster, D. C., Fox, M. L., & Dwyer, D. J. (2001). Explaining employees' health care costs: A prospective examination of stressful job demands, personal control, and physiological reactivity. *Journal of Applied Psychology, 86,* 954–964.

Ghacibeh, G. A., Shenker, J. I., Shenal, B., Uthman, B. M., & Heilman, K. M. (2006). Effect of vagus nerve stimulation on creativity and cognitive flexibility. *Epilepsy & Behavior, 8,* 720–725.

Higgins, E. T. (1996). The "self digest": Self-knowledge serving self-regulatory functions. *Journal of Personality and Social Psychology, 71,* 1062–1083.

Higgins, E. T. (1997). Beyond pleasure and pain. *American Psychologist, 52,* 1280–1300.

Higgins, E. T. (1998). Promotion and prevention: Regulatory focus as a motivational principle. *Advances in Experimental Social Psychology, 30,* 1–46.

Higgins, E. T. (2000). Making a good decision: Value from fit. *American Psychologist, 55,* 1217–1230.

Higgins, E. T., & Tykocinski, O. (1992). Self-discrepancies and biographical memory: Personality and cognition at the level of psychological situation. *Personality and Social Psychology Bulletin, 18,* 527–535.

Izzo, J., L., Levy, D., & Black, H. R. (2000). Importance of systolic blood pressure in older Americans. *Hypertension, 35,* 1021–1024.

Keller, J., & Bless, H. (2006). Regulatory fit and cognitive performance: The interactive effect of chronic and situationally induced self-regulatory mechanisms on test performance. *European Journal of Social Psychology, 36,* 393–405.

Kelsey, R. M., Ornduff, S. R., & Alpert, B. S. (2007). Reliability of cardiovascular reactivity to stress: Internal consistency. *Psychophysiology, 44,* 216–225.

Kristof-Brown, A. L., Zimmerman, R. D., & Johnson, E. C. (2005). Consequences of individuals' fit at work: A meta-analysis of person–job, person–organization, person–group, and person–supervisor fit. *Personnel Psychology, 58,* 281–342.

Larkin, J. E., Pines, H. A., & LaPort, K. A. (2007, March). *Do people "feel right" when experiencing regulatory fit?* Poster session presented at the annual meeting of the Eastern Psychological Association, Philadelphia, PA.

Latimer, A. E., Rivers, S. E., Rench, T. A., Katulak, N. A., Hicks, A., Hodorowski, J. K., . . . Salovey, P. (2008). A field experiment testing the utility of regulatory fit messages for promoting physical activity. *Journal of Experimental Social Psychology, 44,* 826–832.

Llabre, M. M., Spitzer, S. B., Saab, P. G., Ironson, G. H., & Schneiderman, N. (1991). The reliability and specificity of delta versus residualized change as measure of cardiovascular reactivity to behavioral challenges. *Psychophysiology, 28,* 701–711.

Lockwood, P., Jordan, C. H., & Kunda, Z. (2002). Motivation by positive or negative role models: Regulatory focus determines who will best inspire us. *Journal of Personality and Social Psychology, 83,* 854–864.

Matthews, G., Campbell, S. E., Falconer, S., Joyner, L. A., Huggins, J., Gilliland, K., . . . Warm, J. S. (2002). Fundamental dimensions of subjective state performance settings: Task engagement, distress, and worry. *Emotion, 2,* 315–340.

Matthews, G., Joyner, L., Gilliland, K., Campbell, S. Huggins, J., & Falconer, S. (1999). Validation of a comprehensive stress state questionnaire: Towards a state "big three"? In I. Mervielde, I. J. Deary, F. DeFruyt, & F. Ostendorf (Eds.), *Personality Psychology in Europe* (Vol. 7, pp. 335–350). Tilburg, The Netherlands: Tilburg University Press.

O'Donnell, M. P. (2006). Smoke free workplaces: What's the impact on smoking and health? *American Journal of Health Promotion, 20,* iv–v.

Pithers, R. T., & Soden, R. (1999). Person–environment fit and teacher stress. *Educational Research, 41,* 51–61.

Polanyi, M., Frank, J., Shannon, H., Sullivan, T., & Lavis, J. (2000). Promoting the determinants of good health in the workplace. In B. Poland, L. Green,

& I. Rootman (Eds.), *Settings for health promotion: Linking theory and practice* (pp. 138–160). Newbury Park, CA: Sage.

Saks, A. M., & Ashforth, B. E. (1997). A longitudinal investigation of the relationships between job information sources, applicant perceptions of fit, and work outcomes. *Personnel Psychology, 50,* 395–426.

Schmit, M. J., Ryan, A. M., Stierwalt, S. L., & Powell, A. B. (1995). Frame-of-reference effects on personality scale scores and criterion-related validity. *Journal of Applied Psychology, 80,* 607–620.

Schwartz, J. E., Pickering, T. G., & Landsbergis, P. A. (1996). Work-related stress and blood pressure: Current theoretical models and considerations from a behavioral medicine perspective. *Journal of Occupational Health Psychology, 1,* 287–310.

Shah, J., Higgins, E. T., & Friedman, R. S. (1998). Performance incentives and means: How regulatory focus influences goal attainment. *Journal of Personality and Social Psychology, 74,* 285–293.

Sherman, D. K., Bunyan, D. P., Creswell, J. D., & Jaremka, L. M. (2009). Psychological vulnerability and stress: The effects of self-affirmation on sympathetic nervous system responses to naturalistic stressors. *Health Psychology, 28,* 554–562.

Spiegel, S., Grant-Pillow, H., & Higgins, E. T. (2004). How regulatory fit enhances motivational strength during goal pursuit. *European Journal of Social Psychology, 34,* 39–54.

Spokane, A. R., Meir, E. I., & Catalano, M. (2000). Person-environment congruence and Holland's theory: A review and reconsideration. *Journal of Vocational Behavior, 57,* 137–187.

Syme, S. L. (1996). Rethinking disease: Where do we go from here? *Annals of Epidemiology, 6,* 463–468.

Tavares, L. S., & Plotnikoff, R. C. (2008). Not enough time? Individual and environmental implications for workplace physical activity programming among women with and without young children. *Health Care for Women International, 29,* 244–281.

Tinsley, H. E. A. (2000). The congruence myth: An analysis of the person–environment fit model. *Journal of Vocational Behavior, 56,* 147–179.

Wellens, B. T., & Smith, A. P. (2006). Combined workplace stressors and their relationship with mood, physiology, and performance. *Work & Stress, 20,* 245–258.

Westerland, H., Theorell, T., & Alfredsson, L. (2004). Organizational instability and cardiovascular risk factors in white-collar employees. *European Journal of Public Health, 14,* 37–42.

Wright, R. A. (1996). Brehm's theory of motivation as a model of effort and cardiovascular response. In P. M. Gollwitzer & J. A. Bargh (Eds.), *The psychology of action: Linking cognition and motivation to behavior* (pp. 424–453). New York, NY: Guilford Press.

SECTION III

THE ROLE OF THE ORGANIZATION AND QUALITY OF WORK LIFE IN STRESS

CHAPTER 7

THE RELATIONSHIP BETWEEN FAMILY-SUPPORTIVE CULTURE, WORK–FAMILY CONFLICT, AND EMOTIONAL EXHAUSTION

A Multilevel Study

Kristi Zimmerman, Leslie Hammer, and Tori Crain
Portland State University

ABSTRACT

In response to the changes in the composition of families and the workforce, organizations have recognized the need to support employees' work and personal lives in order to minimize negative health and work outcomes associated with experiences of work–family conflict. The primary goal of this chapter is to highlight a study that examines school-level moderating effects of family supportive culture on the relationship between work–family conflict and

Coping and Prevention, pages 111–128

emotional exhaustion in a sample of teachers. Understanding the effects of a family-supportive culture from a multi-level perspective will be an important contribution to the work–family literature.

There is a growing recognition among work–family scholars that organizational context plays an important role in employees' ability to balance work and family (Allen, 2001; Hammer & Zimmerman, 2010; Thompson, Beauvais, & Lyness, 1999). Research generally shows that work–family conflict is significantly correlated with higher work stress, family stress, turnover intentions, and substance abuse, as well as lower family, job, and life satisfaction; organizational commitment and performance (e.g., Allen, Herst, Bruck, & Sutton, 2000; Eby, Casper, Lockwood, Bordeaux, & Brinley, 2005, Kossek & Ozeki, 1998); and higher crossover of work–family conflict among spouses (Hammer, Allen, & Grigsby, 1997). Specific to this study, research has established a significant relationship between work–family conflict and emotional exhaustion such that higher levels of work–family conflict lead to higher levels of emotional exhaustion (e.g., Bacharach, Bamberger, & Conley, 1991; Boles, Johnston, & Hair, 1997; Greenglass & Burke, 1988; Kossek & Ozeki, 1998; Netemeyer, Boles, & McMurrian, 1996; Rupert, Stevanovic, & Hunley, 2009; Yu, Lee, & Tsai, 2010). In addition, the relationship has also been established in teachers, the population of interest in the current study (e.g., Ayo, Henry, & Adebukola, 2009; Innstrand, Langballe, & Falkum, 2010; Papastylianou, Kailia, & Polychronopolous, 2009).

In response conflicting demands between work and family life, many organizations have recognized the need to create family-supportive environments as a way to reduce the negative health and work outcomes associated with conflicts between employees' work and personal lives. Research has reported significant positive relationships between family-supportive culture and job satisfaction and organizational commitment, as well as decreased turnover intentions and work–family conflict (Allen, 2001; Thompson et al., 1999). However, there is minimal research on the effects of a family-supportive culture on burnout/emotional exhaustion with the exception of Cook (2009), who found that family-supportive culture partially mediates the relationship between work–family policies and burnout.

Thus, the primary contributions of this study are: (1) to establish the relationship between work–family conflict and emotional exhaustion in teachers, specifically differentiating between work-to-family and family-to-work conflict; (2) to examine the effects of family-supportive culture at the school level on the relationship between work–family conflict and emotional exhaustion.

This study will draw on work–family research that has examined family-supportive cultures, specifically that of work–family culture (Thompson et al., 1999) and family-supportive organizational perceptions (FSOP) (Allen, 2001). In the following sections, we offer a brief discussion of work–fam-

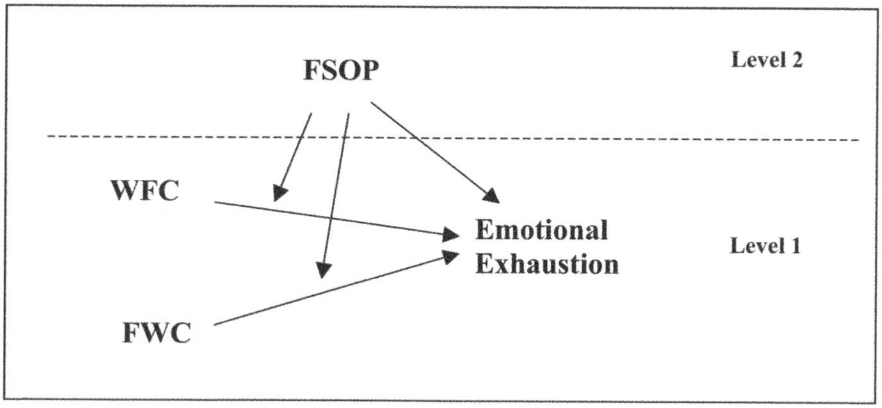

Figure 7.1 Theoretical framework for the relationship between work–family conflict, emotional exhaustion, and family supportive culture.

ily conflict and then move to its role as a predictor of emotional exhaustion. Next, we will turn to a discussion of family-supportive culture as a construct, specifically through discussing the theories of Perceived Organizational Support and Organizational Culture, and emphasizing its role as a cross-level moderator in the current study. The proposed relationships developed in the subsequent sections are depicted in Figure 7.1.

THEORETICAL OVERVIEW OF WORK–FAMILY CONFLICT AND FAMILY-SUPPORTIVE CULTURE

Work–Family Conflict

Work–family conflict is defined as a type of inter-role conflict in which the role demands stemming from one domain (work or family) are incompatible with role demands stemming from the other domain (family or work) (Greenhaus & Beutell, 1985). Work–family conflict originates from the idea of role conflict, which has been defined as the simultaneous occurrence of two or more sets of pressures, such that compliance with one set would make compliance with the other more difficult (Kahn, Wolfe, Quinn, Snoek, & Rosenthal, 1964).

Research in the work–family domain has also emphasized the importance of distinguishing between the two directions of work–family conflict in which work interferes with family (work-to-family conflict) as well as family interferences with work (family-to-work conflict) (Frone, Russell, & Cooper, 1992). Literature suggests that work interference with family may have different antecedents and outcomes than family interference with work (Eby et al., 2005;

Frone, 2003). Frone et al. (1992) tested their model and demonstrated how work-related demands are most often associated with work-to-family conflict and family-related demands are most often associated with family-to-work conflict. That is, stressors in one domain are often related only to same-domain conflict. For example, job stressors were predictive of work-to-family conflict, whereas family stressors and family involvement were predictive of family-to-work conflict (Frone et al., 1992, 1997). However, other researchers (e.g., Grandey & Cropanzano, 1999) have demonstrated how the effects of the conflict can occur in the opposite domain from the originating stressor which is consistent with the spillover model (Kossek & Ozeki, 1998). It is important to recognize that regardless of the direction of the interference, work–family conflict is triggered by simultaneous pressures or demands in both roles (Greenhaus, Allen, & Spector, 2006).

Emotional Exhaustion

It has been commonly assumed that there is something unique about health care, teaching, and other "caring" professions that make their occupants more likely to experience burnout. Burnout has been defined as an affective reaction to stress characterized by depletion over time and consists of three dimensions: emotional exhaustion, depersonalization, and reduced personal accomplishment. This study focuses on the emotional exhaustion component, as it is considered the core component of burnout, and it has been shown that individuals experiencing burnout on the dimension of emotional exhaustion do not necessarily experience the symptoms associated with the dimensions of depersonalization and reduced personal accomplishment (Shirom, 2003). In addition, emotional exhaustion is regarded as the basic individual stress component of the burnout syndrome.

This relationship between work–family conflict and burnout can be examined through the framework of the conservation of resources theory (COR). The COR model proposes that individuals seek to acquire and maintain resources. Stress is a reaction to an environment in which there is the threat of a loss of resources, an actual loss of resources, or lack of an expected gain in resources (Hobfoll, 1989). These resources include objects, conditions, personal characteristics, and energies. When applying COR to work–family conflict, the *conditions* of marital status and tenure are examples of both family and work resources that are valued and sought. *Personal characteristics,* such as self-esteem, are resources that buffer one against stress. *Energies* include resources such as time, money, and knowledge, and they allow one to acquire additional resources (Grandey & Cropanzano, 1999). The COR model proposes that inter-role conflict leads to stress because resources are lost in the process of juggling both work and family roles. As a result of these potential or actual losses of resources, individuals may experience a negative "state of being," which may include dissatisfaction, depression, or anxiety (Grandey & Cropanzano, 1999). It is suggested that some type of behavior, such as planning to leave the work role, is needed to replace or protect the threatened resources. If this type of behavior is not taken, the resources may be so depleted that burnout results.

According to the COR model, as more conflict is experienced in one domain, fewer resources are available to fulfill one's role in another domain. With work-to-family conflict in mind, experiencing high levels of conflict at work might tap available resources and lead to depletion of emotional resources (Grandey & Cropanzano, 1999). Similarly, with family-to-work conflict, experiencing high levels of conflict at home can leave fewer resources available for work demands, leading to this depletion of emotional resources or burnout. Thus, COR theory provides a rationale for examining both work-to-family and family-to-work conflict in relation to burnout.

Empirically, a positive relationship between work–family conflict and burnout has been established (e.g., Bacharach et al., 1991; Greenglass & Burke, 1988; Netemeyer et al., 1996; Kossek & Ozeki, 1999). However, with the exception of a few studies (Lambert, Hogan, & Altheimer, 2010; Yanchus, Eby, Lance, & Drollinger, 2010), most have measured work–family conflict as one construct or they have measured only work-to-family conflict. The current study will separate work-to-family conflict and family-to-work conflict as predictors of emotional exhaustion. Thus:

Hypothesis 1: *Work-to-family conflict is significantly and positively related to emotional exhaustion.*

Hypothesis 2: *Family-to-work conflict is significantly and positively related to emotional exhaustion.*

Family-Supportive Culture

The concept of family-supportive culture originated out of the theories of perceived organizational support and organizational culture. Perceived organizational support (POS) is defined as an employee's global beliefs concerning the extent to which the organization values their contributions and cares about their well-being (Eisenberger, Huntington, Hutchinson, & Sowa, 1986). According to the POS theory, an organization that values the well-being of its employees by showing concern for their needs, goals, and personal problems, also promotes the well-being and health of its personnel. An underlying aspect of POS is organizational culture. Schein (1990) proposed three fundamental levels at which culture manifests itself. The first is the surface level, which includes artifacts that cover everything from the physical layout of the organization to archival signs such as company records and annual reports. The second level includes the kinds of values, strategies, and ideologies that are often clearly spelled out in organizations, forming both official goals for action and performance as well as "ideal worker" characteristics. The third level is comprised of the underlying assumptions, or paradigms, that are taken for granted, determining all perceptions though procedures, feelings, and behavior in the organization (Kinnunen, Mauno, Geurts, Dikkers, 2005).

These three operational levels of organizational culture have been applied to what the work–family literature terms *work–family culture*. According to Lewis (1997), family-friendly policies can be seen as artifacts—that is, surface level indicators or organizational intentions. The second level of work–family culture includes an organization's standards, such as valuing long hours in the workplace, or valuing employees who do not allow family commitments to intrude on their working lives. Finally, at the third level of work–family culture are the organizational actions that might be regarded as indicators of the family-friendly values and assumptions held by that organization (Lewis, 1997). The current study is interested in individual perceptions of organizational support for work and family. Thus, we will focus on the third level of work–family culture.

The Role of Family Supportive Culture in Reducing Work–Family Conflict

Research has found that employees who perceived more supportive work–family cultures were more likely to use work–family benefits than those who perceived less supportive cultures (Thompson et al., 1999). In addition, supportive work–family cultures are shown to be significantly related to affective organizational commitment, turnover intentions, and work-to-family conflict even after controlling for the effects of work–family benefit utilization. Similarly, Allen (2001) found that employees who perceived their organization as more family supportive made greater use of available work–family benefits. Significant main effects between FSOP and several outcome variables showed that employees who perceived their organization as more family supportive experienced less work–family conflict, greater job satisfaction, greater organizational commitment, and fewer turnover intentions than did employees who perceived the organization as less family supportive, even after controlling for benefit availability and managerial support (Allen, 2001).

It is important to note that, to the author's knowledge, none of these studies has examined the moderating effect of a family-supportive culture. However, researchers have found moderating effects for various culture and climate constructs in other realms of organizational research such as organizational safety climate (Probst, 2004). Just as other areas of organizational research have created and tested climate-level variables, we are proposing that work–family research also establish a contextual variable for work–family conflict. We propose that a contextual variable be established in the work–family research for several reasons. First of all, as noted previously, the presence of work–family conflict impairs emotional resources and eventually leads to emotional depletion (Grandey & Cropanzano, 1999). Establishing a family-supportive culture in the workplace would act as a resource to buffer the negative effects experienced from work–family conflict and lead to lower levels of emotional exhaustion. In addition, creating a family-supportive work culture will enable employees to feel more comfortable receiving support and asking for help when situations regarding one's family concerns arise. Finally, research has shown that a family-supportive culture makes employees more likely to use family-friendly policies (Allen, 2001). Thus, family-supportive culture is a contextual variable that will aid in the advancement of the work–family literature in addition to providing various practical implications to organizations. With these arguments in mind, it is proposed that family-supportive culture will interact with work–family conflict such that the relationship between work–family conflict and emotional exhaustion will change depending on the level of family-supportive culture.

In terms of multi-level analyses, we argue that the moderating effect of family-supportive culture represents a "cross-level" process in which a contextual or environmental factor (family-supportive culture) influences the individual-level relationship between work–family conflict and emotional exhaustion. Thus:

> **Hypothesis 3:** *School-level family-supportive culture is a contextual variable that will moderate the relationship between work-to-family conflict and emotional exhaustion. The negative effect of work-to-family conflict on emotional exhaustion will be weaker if there is a high family-supportive culture than if there is a low family-supportive culture.*

> **Hypothesis 4:** *School-level family-supportive culture is a contextual variable that will moderate the relationship between family-to-work conflict and emotional exhaustion. The negative effect of family-to-work conflict on emotional exhaustion will be weaker if there is a high family-supportive culture than if there is a low family-supportive culture.*

METHOD

Participants and Procedures

Participants for the current study were recruited from the 1,250 educators employed by a public school corporation in the U.S. state of Indiana.

Recruitment took place in each of the 33 schools, which include 19 elementary schools, 10 middle schools, and 4 high schools. With a sample size of 850, the response rate was calculated to be 68% with responses from all 33 schools within the district. A 10–15 minute web-based survey was designed to collect desired information from the teachers. Surveys were sent to male and female teachers at all grade levels within the district as well as principals and assistant principals within each school. Teachers were contacted via an email that contained a link to the web-based survey. The association was very interested in implementing family-friendly policies within the schools and sent a flyer to the teachers to encourage participation in the survey. Teachers were also encouraged to complete the survey during work hours. This email was also signed by the teacher's association and the superintendent. In appreciation of their support in completing this survey, the teachers were given the opportunity to enter their email address if they wished to be a part of the drawing for a $100 gift certificate to Target Stores.

Participants were 79% female, and 70% were married with an average of two children. On average, participants had been employed by the school corporation for 14 years, and 72% reported that they were paying members of the teacher's association. Seventy-eight percent of the participants were classified as teachers, with the remaining 22% being administrators, counselors, or other. Average age was 45 years.

Measures

Work–Family Conflict

Work–family conflict was measured with a scale developed by Netemeyer et al. (1996). This measure consists of 10 items to which respondents are to indicate agreement/disagreement on a 5-point scale ranging from 1 (Strongly Disagree) to 5 (Strongly Agree). Five items measure work-to-family conflict (e.g., "The demands of my work life interfere with my family time"). In the current study, Alpha = .91 for work-to-family conflict. In addition, five items measure family-to-work conflict (e.g., "Things I want to do at work don't get done because of the demands of those at home"). In the current study, Alpha = .90 for family-to-work conflict.

Family-Supportive Culture

Family-supportive organization perceptions were measured using Allen's (2001) 9-item scale. This scale asks respondents the degree to which they agree (using a 7-point scale ranging from *strongly disagree* to *strongly agree*) with a series of statements that could describe the philosophy or beliefs of their employing organizations. Higher scores on this scale indicate more family-supportive workplaces. Sample items include, "Expressing involvement and interest in non-work matters is viewed as healthy at my home," and "Employees are given ample opportunity to perform both their job and their personal responsibilities well." In the current study, Alpha = .91 for the construct of family-supportive culture.

Emotional Exhaustion

The emotional exhaustion component of burnout was measured using the Job-Related Exhaustion Scale (Wharton, 1993). The six items refer to the frequency (0 = *never felt this way,* 6 = *felt this way everyday*) of feeling "emotionally drained" and "burned out" from work. Sample items include: "I feel emotionally drained from my work," and "I feel used up at the end of the work day." In the current study, Alpha = .91 for emotional exhaustion.

Control Variables

Possible control variables included marital status, age, number of children living at home, childcare, and paying membership in the teacher's association.

RESULTS

Aggregation

In the current study, Hypotheses 3 and 4 are both cross-level hypotheses in that they involve relationships between family-supportive culture at the school level and work–family conflict and emotional exhaustion at the individual level of analysis. Thus, it was first necessary to make a decision about whether or not the individual-level family-supportive culture data could be aggregated to form school-level values of family-supportive culture. Within group agreement was determined using the Rwg procedure, and results showed that 32 schools displayed an Rwg higher than .70, thus warranting aggregation of individual-level family-supportive culture to the school level.

Multi-Level Modeling

Given the fact that we were interested in modeling the interaction effect of work–family culture (a group-level variable) on an individual-level relationship, the data were analyzed using random coefficient models. Using Mplus, two random coefficient models were estimated for the outcome variable of emotional exhaustion (one model for work-to-family conflict and one model for family-to-work conflict). Family-supportive culture was entered as a Level 2 variable in both models to provide tests of Hypotheses 3 and 4.

Level 1

These random slope models provide tests of Hypotheses 1 and 2 which examined the individual level relationship between work–family (family-to-work) conflict and emotional exhaustion. Specifically, the results of the random slope model with work-to-family conflict as the Level 1 predictor showed a significant main effect for work-to-family conflict on emotional exhaustion and Hypothesis 1 was supported (See Table 7.1). In addition, results for the random coefficient model with family-to-work conflict as the level one predictor showed significant main effect for family-to-work conflict on emotional exhaustion and Hypothesis 2 was supported (See Table 7.2).

Level 2

Hypotheses 3 and 4 examined family-supportive culture as a cross-level moderator to the individual level relationship between work-to-family (family-to-work) conflict and emotional exhaustion. Thus, these hypotheses were also tested with the random coefficient models. However, in order to test for the cross-level moderation, a random slope model was first estimated for the outcome variable of emotional exhaustion in order to ensure that the relationship between work-to-family conflict and emotional exhaustion varied enough across schools to warrant a random coefficient model. These

TABLE 7.1 Random Coefficient Model with WFC Predicting Emotional Exhaustion

Variable	Parameter Estimate	*SE*	Z-ratio	*p*
Within Level				
Gender (β2)	.04	.09	.40	.69
Relationship Status (β3)	.04	.02	1.69	.09
Number of Children at home (β4)	–.06	.03	–2.13	.03
Membership in Teacher's Association (β5)	.04	.06	.06	.58
Within Group Residual for B.O. (V1r*ij*)	.65	.05	14.30	.00
Between Level				
FSOP predicting random slope (γ11)	–.10	.13	–.79	.43
FSOP predicting random intercept (γ01)	–.69	.19	–3.70	.00
Fixed intercept of EE (γ00)	3.13	.04	69.06	.00
Fixed slope of WFC in predicting EE (γ10)	.59	.04	13.31	.00
Between group residual variance for random slope (V1*u*1j)	.01	.02	.76	.22
Between group residual variance for random intercept (V1*u*0j)	.03	.02	1.49	.07

Loglikelihood: H0 = –3573.10

TABLE 7.2 Random Coefficient Model with FWC Predicting Emotional Exhaustion

Variable	Parameter Estimate	*SE*	Z-ratio	*p*
Within Level				
Gender (β2)	.17	.10	1.67	.09
Relationship Status (β3)	.04	.02	1.77	.07
Number of Children at home (β4)	–.09	.03	–2.82	.00
Membership in Teacher's Association (β5)	–.10	.09	–1.24	.21
Within Group Residual for B.O. (V1*rij*)	.86	.05	15.68	.00
Between Level				
FSOP predicting random slope (γ11)	–.10	.39	–.27	.79
FSOP predicting random intercept (γ01)	–.67	.18	–3.65	.00
Fixed intercept of EE (γ00)	3.12	.04	74.24	.00
Fixed slope of WFC in predicting EE (γ10)	.41	.06	6.57	.00
Between group residual variance for random slope (V1*u*1j)	.02	.02	.82	.20
Between group residual variance for random intercept (V1*u*0j)	.01	.01	1.05	.15

Loglikelihood: H0 = –36

analyses were insignificant and indicate that there is not enough variance among schools in terms of their relationships between the work–family variables and emotional exhaustion. Thus, going on to estimate a random coefficient model would not yield a cross-level interaction. This finding indicates that all of the schools had a similar relationship between work-to-family and family-to-work conflict and emotional exhaustion. To ensure the correct results, the necessary analyses were conducted in order to test Hypotheses 3 and 4.

The results of the random coefficient model of work-to-family conflict (Hypothesis 3) indicate that there was no evidence of a cross-level moderation of family-supportive culture on the individual level relationship between work-to-family conflict and emotional exhaustion, and Hypothesis 3 was not supported (see Table 7.1). The results of the random coefficient model for family-to-work conflict (Hypothesis 4) were not significant and indicate no evidence of a cross-level interaction (see Table 7.2). Family-supportive culture at the school level did not moderate the individual level relationship between family-to-work conflict and emotional exhaustion, and Hypothesis 4 was not supported. Finally, the cross-level main effects were examined. Specifically, the effect of school-level family-supportive culture on individual-level emotional exhaustion was observed. The results of the random coefficient model for the cross-level main effects showed a cross-level main effect of group-level family-supportive culture on emotional exhaustion independent of work-to-family conflict. The results for the cross-level main effect for the independent variable of family-to-work conflict showed the presence of a cross-level main effect of group-level family-supportive culture on emotional exhaustion independent of family-to-work conflict. Specifically, increases in school-level family-supportive culture led to decreases in the individual-level burnout regardless of the levels of work-to-family and family-to-work conflict.

DISCUSSION

The results of this study contribute to the work–family literature in a number of ways, as they replicate and extend previous research. Overall, results showed that individual-level work-to-family and family-to-work conflict were significantly related to individual-level emotional exhaustion in teachers. In addition, family-supportive culture at the school level led to decreases in individual levels of emotional exhaustion independent of work-to-family and family-to-work conflict. The significant results of Hypotheses 1 and 2 served to establish a relationship between work-to-family (family-to-work) conflict and emotional exhaustion in a population of teachers. This relationship between work–family conflict and burnout has been previously established (e.g., Bacharach et al., 1991; Greenglass & Burke, 1988; Kossek & Ozeki, 1999) but minimal research (for an exception, see Netemeyer et al., 1996) has examined the bidirectional nature of this relationship, as we did in this study.

Hypotheses 2 and 3 examined family-supportive culture as a cross-level moderator to the individual-level relationship between work–family conflict and emotional exhaustion in teachers. These hypotheses were not supported, as family-supportive culture at the group level was not found to moderate the individual-level relationship between work-to-family (family-to-work) conflict and emotional exhaustion. As noted previously, the insignificant findings resulted from a lack of variance in the individual-level relationship between work–family conflict and emotional exhaustion. A possible explanation for this lack of variance can be understood by looking at the literature that has established this relationship between work–family conflict and emotional exhaustion in teachers. It has consistently been shown that teaching is an occupation that leads to increased levels of burnout and that teachers experiencing a high level of work–family conflict will be burned out (Greenglass & Burke, 1988; Netemeyer et al., 1996). In the current study, 31% of teachers agreed (including agree and strongly agree) to experiencing work–family conflict, and 41% (including agree and strongly agree) of teachers reported burnout. Thus, the lack of variation among schools on individual-level relationships between work–family conflict and burnout may be the result of consistently high levels of work–family conflict and burnout among these teachers. We urge future research to continue to examine family-supportive culture as a moderator of the relationship between work–family conflict and burnout in other occupations where there may be more variance. This null result could also be attributed to possible district-wide effects on the individual schools. Specifically, the policies surrounding work–life balance in this school district are set by the administration, not by the individual schools. For example, the administration decides whether to offer teachers flexible work arrangements or job sharing opportunities, not each individual principal. Thus, in hindsight, work-to-family and family-to-work conflict and their effects on emotional exhaustion may not be expected to vary by school.

Although we did not find a cross-level interaction of family-supportive culture on the relationship between work–family conflict and emotional exhaustion, the multi-level findings still offer several contributions to the work–family literature. Though it was not hypothesized, results indicate a cross-level main effect of family-supportive culture on emotional exhaustion for the independent variables of work-to-family and family-to-work conflict. That is, increases in group-level family-supportive culture resulted in decreases in levels of emotional exhaustion independent of work-to-family (family-to-work conflict) in teachers. This finding indicates that school-level family-supportive culture reduces levels of emotional exhaustion that are not necessarily experienced as a result of work-to-family or family-to-work conflict. It is possible that a supportive culture in general can lead to decreases in emotional exhaustion regardless of what the focus of the support may be. Turning again to the COR model, this finding shows that schools can offer teacher resources that may decrease emotional exhaustion that is experienced as a result of other stressors aside from work–family conflict. For instance, health-related stressors may be alleviated by school-specific wellness programs.

On another note, this finding indicates that individual perceptions of family-supportive culture do in fact cluster to form a group-level construct. This lends support to the idea of using family-supportive culture as a group-level variable in future research. Just as safety climate has been established as a multi-level variable in the safety research (e.g., Probst, 2004; Hoffman, Morgeson, & Gerras, 2003), family-supportive culture could serve as an important multi-level variable in future work–family research.

This finding also supports the idea of using multi-level modeling to examine occupational stress outcomes (e.g., emotional exhaustion). Like most phenomena studied in the organizational sciences, it is understood that the study of occupational stress is best approached from a multilevel perspective (Klein, Dansereau, & Hall, 1994). Thus, understanding both individual differences (e.g., work–family conflict) and contextual effects of environmental differences (e.g., school family-supportive culture) can serve to enhance our theoretical understanding of occupational stress.

Implications

This study offers several practical implications in addition to the theoretical advancements. Modeling the contextual effects of family-supportive culture may have considerable practical significance in occupational stress research and practice. The presence or absence of contextual effects has important implications for designing and implementing interventions (Jex & Bliese, 1999). In cases where stressors and strains do not cluster by group, individual-based intervention strategies may be the most effective means of reducing this work stress. In contrast, if stressors and strains cluster by group, this indicates that there is some aspect of the environment distinct from the attributes of the individuals that is related to the outcome (Jex & Bliese, 1999). In these cases, intervention strategies may be most effective if directed at groups.

Specific to the current study, the main group-level effect of family-supportive culture on emotional exhaustion indicates that group-level family-supportive culture was significantly related to individual-level reports of emotional exhaustion such that higher levels of family-supportive culture led to lower levels of emotional exhaustion. Therefore, in this case an intervention to decrease levels of emotional exhaustion should be focused at the school level. For example, 63% of participants in the current study indicated interest in stress reduction programs and 41% of teachers expressed interest in work–family informational seminars. In addition, 62% reported that they would take advantage of flexible work hours if the option were available. Thus, administration may seek to enforce stronger implementation of these types of policies and programs in those schools exhibiting high levels of emotional exhaustion.

Creating a more family-supportive culture for teachers will help to lower levels of burnout and thus increase job satisfaction and productivity. It is important to look at levels of burnout in teachers due to the fact that burned-out employees have been shown to be less productive to their organization (Kossek & Ozeki, 1999). Emotional exhaustion has been linked to several negative organizational outcomes including increased turnover and absenteeism as well as lower organizational commitment (e.g., Jackson, Schwab, & Schuler, 1986). In addition, teachers hold a lot of responsibility as they are educating the future minds of America, and if teachers come to work burnt out, children may not be receiving the best possible education. A significant relationship between school-level family-supportive culture and emotional exhaustion is an important sign for administrators to think about ways to create a more family-supportive workplace in order to reduce teacher burnout and decrease the attrition rates among educators.

Limitations and Future Research

The main limitation of the current study is the cross-sectional design. Although the path models in this study showed which direction of the relationship between work–family conflict and emotional labor best fit our data, causal relationships could not be generalized to other studies. Future research should use a longitudinal design in order to establish these causal relationships. In addition, although controlled for in all analyses, the fact that 80% of the respondents were female may also limit how well the results would generalize to a more heterogeneous population. The self-report nature of my data collection presents another limitation. Due to the fact that teachers could choose what questions they wanted to answer in the survey, many questions were left unanswered, resulting in missing data.

Another limitation to this study is the possibility of district-wide effects on the individual-level relationships. We found that the relationship between work–family conflict and emotional exhaustion did not vary by schools. It is possible that this could be due to the fact that the family-friendly policies (or lack thereof) are district-wide policies rather than policies specific to individual schools, which may explain why this work–family conflict-emotional exhaustion relationship did not vary by schools.

This study offers several directions for future research. As mentioned previously, multi-level modeling is a key way to model contextual effects within organizations. Bliese and Jex (2002) suggest more research along the lines of this study is needed that incorporates a multi-level perspective into research on occupational stress. Furthermore, Klein and colleagues have been arguing for multilevel organizational research to capture the true relationships in such structures (Klein, Tosi, & Cannella, 1999). The main cross-level effect of family-supportive culture in the current study encourages more research to explore this variable as a multi-level construct. We suggest testing family-supportive culture in other occupations that may not have the district-wide effects that exist in education. In general, this study paves the way for more multilevel research to be done in the realm of work and family.

CONCLUSION

The findings of this research contribute to the work–family field in a number of ways. The primary goal of this study was to examine the cross-level moderating effects of family-supportive culture on the relationship between work–family conflict and emotional exhaustion. Although we did not find a significant interaction, the results of the multi-level modeling suggests many directions for future research. Finding a cross-level main effect of family-supportive culture on emotional exhaustion is an important sign that this culture does exist within schools, and low levels of it will lead to increased emotional exhaustion. This stresses the practical importance of implementing family-supportive policies and programs in order to minimize levels of burnout in teachers.

REFERENCES

Allen, T. D. (2001). Family-supportive work environments: The role of organizational perceptions. *Journal of Vocational Behavior, 58,* 414–435.

Allen, T. D., Herst, D. E., Bruck, C.S., & Sutton, M. (2000). Consequences associated with work-to-family conflict: A review and agenda for future research. *Journal of Occupational Health Psychology,* 5, 278–308.

Ayo, H. T., Henry, A. S., & Adebukola T. (2009). Psychosocial variables as predictors of work–family conflict among secondary school teachers in Irele local government area, Ondo State, Nigeria. *Pakistan Journal of Social Sciences, 6*(1), 11–18.

Bacharach, S.B., Bamberger, P., Conley, S. (1991). Work–home conflict among nurses and engineers: Mediating the impact of role stress on burnout and satisfaction at work. *Journal of Organizational Behavior, 12,* 39–53.

Bliese, P. D., & Jex, S. M. (2002). Incorporating a multilevel perspective into occupational stress research: Theoretical, methodological, and practical implications. *Journal of Occupational Health Psychology,* 7(3), 265–276.

Boles, J.S., Johnston, M.W., & Hair, J.F. (1997). Role stress, work–family conflict and emotional exhaustion: Inter-relationships and effects on some work-related consequences. *Journal of Personal Selling and Sales Management, 27,* 17–28.

Cook, A. (2009). Connecting work–family policies to supportive work environments. *Group and Organizational Management, 34*(2), 206–240.

Eby, L. T., Casper, W., Lockwood, A., Bordeaux, C., & Brinley, A. (2005). A twenty year retrospective on work and family research in IO/OB journals: A review of the literature. *Journal of Vocational Behavior, Monograph, 66,* 124–197.

Eisenberger, R., Huntington, R., Hutchison, & S. Sowa, D. (1986). Perceived organizational support. *Journal of Applied Psychology, 71,* 500–507.

Frone, M.R. (2003). Work–family balance. In J. C. Quick & L. E. Tetrick (Eds.), *Handbook of occupational health psychology* (pp. 143–162). Washington, DC: American Psychological Association.

Frone, M. R., Russell, M., & Cooper, M. L. (1992). Antecedents and outcomes of work–family conflict: Testing a model of the work–family interface. *Journal of Applied Psychology, 77,* 65–78.

Frone, M. R., Russell, M., & Cooper, M. L. (1997). Relation of work–family conflict to health outcomes: A four-year longitudinal study of employed parents. *Journal of Occupational and Organizational Psychology, 70,* 325–335.

Grandey, A. A., & Cropanzano, R. (1999). The conservation of resources model applied to work–family conflict and strain. *Journal of Vocational Behavior, 54*(2), 350–370.

Greenglass, E. R., & Burke, R. J. (1988). Work and family precursors of burnout in teachers: Sex differences. *Sex Roles, 18,* 215–229.

Greenhaus, J. H., Allen, T. D., & Spector, P. E. (2006). Health consequences of work–family conflict: The dark side of the work–family interface. In P.L. Perrewé & D.C. Ganster (Eds.), *Research in occupational stress and well-being* (pp. 61–98). JAI Press/Elsevier.

Greenhaus, J. H., & Beutell, N. J. (1985). Sources of conflict between work and family roles. *Academy of Management Review, 10,* 76–88.

Hammer, L., Allen, E., & Grigsby, T. (1997). Work–family conflict in dual-earner couples: Within-individual and crossover effects of work and family. *Journal of Vocational Behavior, 50,* 185–203.

Hammer, L. B., & Zimmerman, K. L. (2011). Quality of work life. In S. Zedeck (Ed.), *American Psychological Association handbook of industrial and organizational psychology* (Vol. 3., pp. 399–431). Washington, DC: American Psychological Association.

Hobfoll, S. E. (1989). Conservation of resources: A new attempt at conceptualizing stress. *American Psychologist, 44,* 513–524.

Hoffman, D. A., Morgeson, F. P., & Gerras, S. J. (2003). Climate as a moderator of the relationship between leader–member exchange and content specific citizenship: Safety climate as an exemplar. *Journal of Applied Psychology, 88,* 170–178.

Innstrand, S. T., Langballe, E.M., & Falkum, E. (2010). Exploring occupational differences in work–family interaction: Who is at risk? *International Journal of Stress Management, 17*(1), 38–55.

Jackson, S. E., Schwab, R. L., & Schuler, R. S. (1986). Toward an understanding of the burnout phenomenon. *Journal of Applied Psychology, 71,* 630–640.

Jex, S. M., & Bliese, P. D. (1999). Efficacy beliefs as a moderator of the impact of work-related stressors: A multilevel study. *Journal of Applied Psychology, 84*(3), 349–361.

Kahn, R. L., Wolfe, D. M., Quinn, R., Snoek, J. D., & Rosenthal, R. A. (1964). *Organizational Stress.* New York: Wiley.

Kinnunen, U., Mauno, S., Geurts, S., & Dikkers, J. (2005). Work–family culture in organizations: Theoretical and empirical approaches. In S. Poelmans (Ed). *Work and family: An international research perspective* (pp. 87–120). Mahwah, NJ: Lawrence Erlbaum Associates.

Klein, K. J., Dansereau, F., & Hall, R. J. (1994). Levels issues in theory development, data collection, and analysis. *Academy of Management Review, 19*(2), 195–229.

Klein, K. J., Tosi, H., & Cannella, A. A., Jr. (1999). Multilevel theory building: Benefits, barriers, and new developments. *Academy of Management Review, 24*(2), 243–248.

Kossek. E. E., & Ozeki, C. (1998). Work–family conflict, policies, and the job–life satisfaction relationship: A review and directions for organizational behavior/ human resources research. *Journal of Applied Psychology, 83,* 139–149.

Kossek, E. E., & Ozeki, C. (1999). Bridging the work–family policy and productivity gap. *International Journal of Community, Work, and Family, 2*(1), 7–32.

Lambert, E., Hogan, N. L., & Altheimer, I. (2010). The association between work–family conflict and job burnout among correctional staff: A preliminary study. *American Journal of Criminal Justice, 35,* 37–55.

Lewis, S. (1997). Family friendly employment policies: A route to changing organizational culture or playing about at the margins. *Gender, Work and Organization, 4,* 13–23.

Netemeyer, R. G., Boles, J. S., & McMurrian, R. (1996). Development and validation of work–family conflict and family-work conflict scales. *Journal of Applied Psychology, 81,* 400–410.

Papastylianou, A., Kailia, M., & Polychronopolous, M. (2009). Teacher's burnout, depression, role ambiguity and conflict. *Social Psychological Education, 12,* 295–314.

Probst, T.M. (2004). Safety and insecurity: Exploring the moderating effect of organizational safety climate. *Journal of Occupational Health Psychology, 9,* 3–10.

Rupert, P. A., Stevanovic, P., & Hunley, H. A. (2009). Work–family conflict and burnout among practicing psychologists. *Professional Psychology: Research and Practice, 40*(1), 54–61.

Schein, E. (1990). Organizational Culture. *American Psychologist, 45,* 109-119.

Shirom, A. (2003). Job-related burnout. In J. C. Quick & L. E. Tetrick (Eds.), *Handbook of occupational health psychology* (pp. 245–265). Washington, DC: American Psychological Association.

Thompson, C. A., Beauvais, L. L., & Lyness, K. S. (1999). When work–family benefits are not enough: The influence of work–family culture on benefit utilization, organizational attachment, and work–family conflict. *Journal of Vocational Behavior, 54,* 392–415.

Yanchus, N. J., Eby, L. T., Lance, C. E., & Drollinger, S. (2010). The impact of emotional labor on work–family outcomes. *Journal of Vocational Behavior, 76,* 105–117.

Yu, M., Lee, Y., & Tsai, B. (2010). Relationships among stressors, work–family conflict, and emotional exhaustion: A study of the electronics industry employees in China. *Social Behavior and Personality, 38*(6), 829–844.

Wharton, A. S. (1993). The affective consequences of service work. *Work and Occupations, 20,* 205–232.

CHAPTER 8

STRESS MANAGEMENT AND OCCUPATIONAL QUALITY OF LIFE PROGRAMS IN PUBLIC SECURITY

Tatiana Severino de Vasconcelos
University of Brasília

Starting in June 2000, with the launch of the National Public Security Plan and the establishment of the National Public Security Fund, the Federal Administration took an important step in the management of the Brazilian public security system. Among the principles of the National Public Security System we can highlight the following: Human Rights and law enforcement efficiency are compatible and mutually necessary; law enforcement officers are human beings, workers and citizens, and they have rights and privileges given to them by the constitution. Among the targets for the establishment of the principles we may highlight the following: promote a greater respect to the laws and human rights (including by law enforcement officers), improve law enforcement efficiency and fight corruption and violence by police officers and, finally, value the police force and police officers, reforming institutions and training police officers, making people once again trust them and reducing the life risk they are subjected to.

Coping and Prevention, pages 129–145

With the advent of the new National Public Security Plan for Brazil, in 2003, advances were made in Public Security and the United Public Security System was designed and implemented—SUSP in its Portuguese acronym. The purpose of this system is to bring together federal, state, and local actions in public security and criminal justice in order to integrate them in practice, without interfering with the autonomy of their respective agencies. The new plan includes programs linked to two sets of guidelines: (1) programs to reform law enforcement agencies, and (2) violence-reduction programs.

The first set of programs includes public policies designed to improve the image and train law enforcement officer, knowledge management, institutional reorganization, modernization of investigation, bringing together integrated social actions by civil society organizations and the external control of police forces (IPEA, 2003).

According to this new Public Security paradigm, law enforcement officers would no longer take isolated actions that identify citizens as potential enemies, admitting now that in a democratic society public security can only work if it operates in connection with organized communities. The meaning of citizen security is materialized through partnerships between law enforcement agencies and communities in the assessment, planning, and control of interventions.

In 2007, an additional instrument was launched to strengthen the guidelines proposed by the SUSP, the National Program of Security with Citizens' Participation (PRONASCI), made up of four axes: training of law enforcement officers and appreciation of the work they do, restructuring of the prison system, fight against police corruption, and community involvement in violence prevention. The program includes a direct investment by the federal administration of R$ 6,707 billion until 2012.

Therefore, what the National Public Security Plan and its actions stress is the fact that a new public security concept cannot be fully implemented without turning the attention to the issue of human capital. In order for this new concept to become fully effective, it is imperative and urgent that professional qualification measures are taken, not only for continuous training, such as the National Network for Higher Studies in Public Security (RENAESP), the establishment of the security-related technology axis, and the inclusion of higher education programs of Technology in Public Security, in Criminal Services and in Traffic Security in the National Registry of Higher Education Technology Program of the Brazilian Ministry of Education (MEC). These measures undoubtedly represent great steps for the construction of knowledge in the specific field of public security and for the continuous education of law enforcement officers who are more critical, better prepared, and, consequently, more secure regarding the professional activities they have to perform and their interaction with the community.

Nevertheless, adverse work conditions, the risks inherent in the profession, the extenuating work days and the pressure for efficiency made by society expose these professionals to occupational diseases, high stress levels, wear and psychological distress. The concept of risk plays a key role in work, environmental and relational conditions for the profession because its members are constantly exposed and their spirits can never rest (Souza & Minayo, 2005). Therefore, professional qualification measures should urgently comprehend the establishment of better work conditions, illness prevention and promotion of quality of life.

OCCUPATIONAL STRESS

Surprisingly, most people easily say they are stressed, but they have difficulty clearly defining what stress is. In fact, the stress experience or perception can vary from individual to individual, but its effects can be clearly seen in activities such as those of public security professionals. One of the most common presentations is the high percentage of drinking-related problems among police officers when compared to the general population (Glenn et al., 2003). However, there is a scarcity of scientific information on occupational stress, which makes it difficult to properly describe the specific elements of the job that cause stress responses. This means that defining the cause of stress becomes very complex, involving the work environment, the individual, and factors external to work (Stacciarini & Trócolli, 2000).

There are several definitions for this phenomenon, but, generally speaking, all of them are related to the excess of stimuli or demands individuals have difficulties properly coping with and responding to. Studies on occupational stress have also included personality variables, coping, and satisfaction. Occupational stress consists of a perception characterized by ambiguity, conflict, and overload resulting from characteristics both from the individual and the organization (Tetrick, 1992). There are many situations that contribute to the experience of occupational stress, among them role ambiguity and conflict, not enough activities, overload of functions, and responsibility by other people (Dobreva-Martinova, Villeneuve, Strickland, & Matheson, 2002). These forms of stress can lead to poor performance at work (Babin & Boles, 1996) and job dissatisfaction (Hughes, 2001), in addition to being related to poorer health and well-being outcomes (Jones, Flynn, & Kelloway, 1995).

The physical presentations of stress usually include tremors, sweating, increased heart rate, and high blood pressure, among others (Inglehart, 1991). Symptom progression, in the most serious cases, can lead, particularly in public security officers, to problems of substance abuse, violence, despair, and, in extreme circumstances, to suicide.

Stress among Public Security Workers

Data from research studies related to work conditions, mortality, and victimization among public security professionals in Brazil, specifically in Rio de Janeiro, show that the average number of sick leave days among military police officers increased around 95% during the study period (2000–2004), whereas the number of sick leave days among corporals, the frontline officers facing confrontations, more than doubled, reaching 108% (Souza & Minayo, 2005). Regarding partial physical disabilities (PPD), the average number of officers with injuries and traumas increased 166.5% in the period and that of corporals increased 227.5%. Police victimization as a whole, for city guards and civil and military police officers, increased in the study period, as did the number of criminal cases in the state of Rio de Janeiro. However, we should highlight the high victimization rates while these officers were on their day off, which can be attributed to two factors: the high number of police officers who work as private security guards and their involvement in conflicts in neighborhoods, bars, and public transportation vehicles. Additionally, they also fall victim to ambush by criminals, which makes police officers hide their professional identities for their own protection (Souza & Minayo, 2005).

STRATEGIES TO IMPLEMENT THE NATIONAL HEALTHCARE AND QUALITY OF LIFE PROJECT FOR PUBLIC SECURITY OFFICERS

The quality of life concept includes multidimensional and subjective factors related to the individual perception people have about different factors related not only to their physical and psychological health, but also to cultural, time, social, economic and political aspects. Quality of life at the workplace, in turn, comprises two interdependent perspectives. According to Ferreira (2006), from the point of view of leaders and managers, it is an organizational management principle that includes standards, guidelines, and practices designed to promote both individual and collective well-being, the personal development of workers, and the exercise of organizational citizenship. From the point of view of workers, it consists of the representations they build of the organization where they work, indicating the kind of well-being experiences they have at work, the recognition they get from the organization and their coworkers, the possibility of professional growth, and respect to individual characteristics.

In order to encourage and implement effective actions to decrease the vulnerability of public security agents, the National Department of Public Security with the Ministry of Justice (Secretaria Nacional de Seguranca Publica—SENASP, 2006) has established the Coordination of the Quality of Life Project for Public Security Officers, which is designed to plan, implement, follow, and assess policies aimed at promoting the quality of life of these workers. The first step taken in 2008 at the federal administration level for the implementation of policies related to health, quality of life, and stress prevention among the above-mentioned workers was a national Survey of Healthcare and Quality of Life Programs at State Public Security Organizations. Data were collected in eighteen Brazilian states and at the federal district in the five Brazilian regions. The main purpose was to identify projects related to quality of life and collective health, the methods used, and the structures in place in order to get information to design a national policy related to this issue.

The general results showed 96.2% of the organizations surveyed had some kind of healthcare program for their employees. Although there were initiatives of biopsychosocial programs in most states, qualitative reports show that many improvements have to be made and more support has to be given so that these projects can become more effective. In most states, programs have not been officially regulated yet, thus leading to instability of the actions. Additionally, there is a serious lack of human resources and infrastructure, if we consider that many public security organizations do not have their own healthcare professionals and the healthcare services operate in poor conditions. Therefore, when there is a change in management, often the current program is interrupted and actions are discontinued. Another serious problem is the lack of a formal mapping of the problems to decide which action strategies will be implemented, as well as insufficient assessment of the impact and effects once actions are taken. Actions are mostly focused on treating problems that already exist through individual medical treatment or other palliative measures, at the expense of prevention, health, and quality of life promotion activities.

However, in spite of all the problems and needs pointed out by the 2008 survey, it revealed several successful actions and programs in some organizations that could be replicated elsewhere or that could be further encouraged so that they could reach a larger number of workers. In this context, the idea of publishing a quality of life guide directed to the implementation of biopsychosocial care actions emerged. The guide was published by SENASP in March 2010 and is divided into four areas: Human Resources and Material Management, Access to Healthcare and Health Maintenance, Support to Public Security Workers and Their Families, and Strengthening of the Institutional Image. For every action proposed, it presents the context, the main items to be developed, suggestions made by departments and professional in charge, their integration with other actions, the main performance indicators, and benchmark actions found in the surveyed organizations.

By understanding stress and quality of life as multidimensional concepts, we understand that all actions proposed by the guide, to a greater or lesser degree, work as health and well-being promoters, either for already existing diseases or conditions, minimizing the effects of stress, or preventing their occurrence.

Therefore, the guide should serve as a reference source and a "database of ideas" to design actions related to quality of life, showing what are the benchmark projects so that readers could search for additional information and put together similar measures in their own organizations.

Additionally, in order to standardize the implementation of actions and strengthen a national policy regarding this subject, in July 2009 SENASP established a working group (WG) to draft the guidelines for a national project. In order for the project to take the needs of the target audience into account, the WG was composed of healthcare managers from all Brazilian states and the federal district, in addition to representatives from the federal police department and the special human rights department. Out of the discussions held by the group came the Normative Guideline GAB MJ 01/2010, drafted by the whole group, which establishes the project quality of life of public security officers and prison officers. It is designed to foster, in the Brazilian states that voluntarily join the project, preventive and integrated actions in order to prevent illness and promote better living and work conditions for these individuals. The normative guideline is organized in chapters that include certain structures and programs in the participating organizations such as:

- Establishment of an Integrated Healthcare Management Committee for Law Enforcement Officers (CGIAS), made up of healthcare managers from all local law enforcement organizations
- Implementation of Integrated Rehabilitation and Readaptation Centers (CIRR) designed to rehabilitate workers, particularly those injured in the line of duty
- Establishment of Integrated Centers for Biopsychosocial Care (NIAB) that would be in charge of carrying out the quality of life actions in every institution, including preventive activities, decreasing risks, health promotion, and various services
- Continuously see to the rights of public security officers and prison officers
- Establishment of regular tests for prevention purposes and to follow the health indicators of law enforcement officers
- Care of those involved in critical incidents or risk events—organize a specific program for the prevention of post-traumatic stress disorder (PTSD)

- Standardize physical activities and occupational exercise and encourage the activities included in the National Policy of Integrated and Complementary Practices of the Public Healthcare System.

Both the actions guide and the Normative Guideline 01/10 outline extensive and comprehensive health promotion and quality of life programs. However, we must go deeper into the details of actions, the operational mode, and how to learn from successful experiences. Additionally, there are plans to extend and deepen the guide actions through specific working groups, trainin,g and support to state-level projects.

An important component of the support to state-level projects was funding with federal resources, in December 2008, for the implementation of the Integrated Center for Stress Prevention and Management in ten Brazilian states. The ten projects to implement the centers were completed in December 2010 and, generally speaking, presented positive results. Nine states out of ten managed to implement all the project targets, which basically consisted of (1) physical structuring of the Integrated Center for Stress Prevention and Management through the acquisition of fixed assets, supplies, books and films; (2) contracting, for 12 months, of specialized staff for the center and for care provision, such as psychologists, social workers, psychiatrists, physical therapists, occupational physicians, and others; (3) contracting a company to survey the sources and levels of stress of law enforcement officers; (4) educational campaigns and workshops based on survey results; (5) training the healthcare and people management teams in the participating institutions on the subject of stress. The plan is to bring together in one single document the results of this survey that will be carried out independently in the nine states that meet this target in order to guide future actions. Preliminary analyses show that among the most significant sources of stress for these professionals are the following: not being properly appreciated by society, lack of institutional support, lack of equipment, death of colleagues or people they could not save, and insufficient training. These results show the need to invest in preventive programs and the need to rethink the management of public security institutions—that is, to act at the source of the psychological distress, which is related to performance, which is mainly related to organizational and structural issues.

Although organizational factors constitute sources of stress, we cannot ignore the individual component as key in the process, particularly in the area of public security, where individual resistance to pressure and the way individuals can cope with the problems and risks inherent in the profession are also determining factors. In this regard, the psychological assessment during selection processes is a key to selecting individuals who are better able to carry out the tasks demanded from their job, in addition to trying to exclude those who have psychological conditions that are incompatible with their job. In spite of the importance of a proper psychological assessment, based on an occupational profile, public security institutions not always have such a formal document or use scientifically built profiles. The job design used today often does not take into account factors such as knowledge, skills, and attitudes required to carry out tasks and a description of obstacles and facilitating factors (organizational support). In other cases, the job description is made empirically, based solely on the opinion of managers and supervisors, without taking into account the actual activities performed by workers. Additionally, there is no formal diagnosis or survey of the training needs that would enable a proper planning of the management actions of the institutions, such as team building, selection, job assessment, performance appraisal, training planning, citizen services, management and professional development, counseling, career development, leadership development, and conflict management. The lack of a formal definition for the job profiles can result in difficulties in team management, communication problems, inadequate selection, overload of activities and mismatch between prescribed and actual work, generating uncertainties and impacting the performance of activities at the organization, that is, it becomes one additional source of occupational stress.

Considering the above, SENASP acted on two different fronts:

- Signing of agreements with six states to make occupational profiles and survey of skills required for the jobs of soldier and lieutenant of the military police and the military fire department and the jobs of civil police agent and chief police officer, in addition to training of the management professionals in the training course Occupational Profiling Methodology and Skills Survey
- Occupational Profiling National Survey: the survey is being conducted in partnership with the United Nations Development Program (UNDP) to survey information that will make up an occupational profile of the professionals working at the public security state organizations (i.e., civil police, military police, and military fire department) and the respective mapping of the skills required to perform their activities, identifying, comparing, and establishing the common/different set of knowledge, skills, and attitudes that make up the occupational profile of public security professionals.

Occupational profiling is a method used to get to know more deeply the types of jobs, the morphological-physical-psychological requirements for their performance, and the fit between worker/job/work environment and the goals to be achieved: productivity, accident prevention, and the preservation of workers' health and physical integrity. Its product is the detailed analysis of the job, showing its mission, the tasks to be performed, the facilitating factors, obstacles, and requirements. The knowledge of the occupational profile and the identification of the common features of public security workers who work in this context will contribute to the effectiveness of the results of the training actions that are jointly planned and carried out.

Competence mapping, on the other hand, consists of identifying the competences professionals have and what their gaps are in order to optimize their performance in addition to making them realize they need to look for their self-development. The competence mapping process enables us to more efficiently find what the training needs are, because it shows what the proposed competences or skills are that the professional should acquire. Therefore, aligning the individual competences of their professionals with those required to achieve their strategic objectives is an important step to reform law enforcement agencies. The survey reached 3,782 respondents at the Military Fire Department, 24,678 at the Military Police, and 5,432 at the Civil Police, and their results will contribute to improve and update the National Curriculum for the Training of Public Security Professionals.

In addition to the previously mentioned strategies, it is also fundamental to conduct specific research to investigate the factors that lead to disease and to poorer work conditions of public security agents. In this regard, information collection is an important tool for decision-making, design of healthcare public policies and the implementation of the National Quality of Life Project for Public Security Workers. It is necessary to investigate the relationship between work conditions, specifically the different working hour schemes, the sickness pattern, and sick leave days taken by the officers. The results of the investigation should identify the sources and causes of the problems found at the institutions, thus enabling them to adopt preventive and treatment actions. There is still an intense debate in public security surrounding the different working hour schemes: how appropriate they are and their implications for management. We also have to take into account the impact of the different working hour schemes on the quality of life of these workers, on their family and social relationships, on their leisure activities, and on their health as a whole. Different states regulate the working hours of public security agents differently, the most common schemes being 24 hours of work followed by 48 hours off, 24 × 72 hours, or even alternate schemes of 12 × 24 and 12 × 48. However, the discussion around what should be the most appropriate working hour scheme has not been based on scientific evidence considering the actual implications of working hours on the administrative management of the corporation and on the health and quality of life of the workers.

Therefore, SENASP realized they had to conduct a survey to map working conditions and hours and their implications on the health of public security workers, which is currently in the planning phase. The results of this survey will be fundamental for the implementation of new guidelines and policies for the National Quality of Life Project and also to cast light on and serve as a foundation for the debate on the different working hours schemes that currently exist. Additionally, survey results will be an indispensable source of information for the planning, follow-up, and assessment of public security policies implemented at the local and regional level, particularly those designed to promote the quality of life and to prevent sickness and psychological distress among law enforcement officers.

Another gap that has been identified that impacts the implementation of quality of life projects is the disconnection and poor communication among institutions. The establishment of such programs, particularly in public service, should be based on the synergism among people and exchange of information and experiences among institutions. In this regard, with the support of SENASP and the participation of all Brazilian public security institutions the Quality of Life Network for Public Security was established and regulated on May 24, 2010 through Order MJ no. 14. The objective is to establish and organize a collaborative network where the best practices in the area of biopsychosocial care can be disseminated and shared, aiming at a greater integration among the different institutions. The representatives from the different institutions participating in the network are appointed by the leaders of every institution and should be strategic managers in healthcare and/or people management. All appointees should be registered in an internet-based system that will be accessed by everybody and that will enable fast communication. Among the main activities carried out by network members are the contact with SENASP and other institutions, supporting research work, encouraging educational and awareness campaigns, participation in training actions promoted and supported by SENASP, and supporting the proposal of public policies designed to provide better biopsychosocial care, among others.

Regarding the thematic working groups, a first WG was established in December 2010 to discuss the impact of personal protective equipment (PPE) and collective protective equipment (CPE) on workers' health and performance. This first WG focused on military police officers, considering the fact that they represent the largest number of police officers in Brazil. The purpose of the WG, which gathered experts and technicians from military police departments from all over Brazil, in addition to members of the civil police, the fire department and the ministry of labor, was to increase the knowledge about legislation on the subject, material specifications, impacts of wearing/not wearing protective equipment, training needs, and protective equipment management policies. The discussion coming out of the WG will result in a standard at the federal government level with guidelines related to the purchase of PPE and CPE, making sure that new equipment purchase projects are mandatorily connected to training, risk and accident prevention, and professional qualification actions.

EXPERIENCES IN OTHER COUNTRIES

Based on the survey of good practices in Brazil in the area of healthcare and qualification of law enforcement workers, we once again turn our attention to successful experiences in other countries. Abroad, particularly in the United States, great attention is given to the care given to public security workers after critical events, such as events involving confrontation with fire weapons; witnessing death, suicide, or other great tragedies; and risks to the physical, psychological, and moral integrity of law enforcement workers. Another major focus of studies and scientific research has been the effectiveness of psychosocial programs or services.

Considering that police officers are often exposed to high-stress situations, assessing the individual differences in their response patterns is of paramount importance. Research studies in this area aim to clarify this issue and help managers to understand the trauma and stress response patterns, the connection between trauma and substance abuse, and the intervention and treatment strategies that are required to help public security workers survive the hardships of their profession.

The predictors of psychological distress among police officers have been extensively investigated in other countries. Wang et al. (2010) found that depression predictors include major childhood trauma, lower self-esteem during the training program, and greater perception of stress in the first year of work. Knowing the predictors is important for the identification, whenever possible, of the most vulnerable individuals. However, in practice this identification has only been possible at the time of the psychological assessment made before people can join a public security institution. It is therefore crucial to outline the profile required for every job, make a thorough psychological assessment, and turn away those applicants who represent a potential risk for themselves and for other people if they are to work as law enforcement officers.

In addition to the recruitment assessment, applicants should be closely followed during their training courses in order to check how they respond to the pressures of the profession, to the interaction with their colleagues, and to the contact with the culture of the institution. Therefore, ideally they should undergo a psychological assessment throughout their training period, not only before they join the institution. These findings reinforce the importance of investigating the personal features that influence performance as well as the appropriate personnel selection techniques. In order for this to happen, (1) valid and reliable instruments must be developed to assess the individual features of the applicants, such as personality traits, coping skills, reasoning, specific skills, and (2) research should be conducted showing the importance and predictive ability of these individual features. In other words, good psychological assessment instruments are required for reliable predictive assessment to be made, because the former would have been based on studies that considered concrete function performances (Vasconcelos, 2005). Regarding the specific activities performed by law enforcement officers, the literature highlights the importance of adaptive behaviors; that is, many of the activities carried out by police officers show that the ability to adapt to extreme, unexpected, and emergency situations is a crucial characteristic and one that can predict the long-term effectiveness of the organization (Hackett, 2002).

RESPONSE TO PROBLEMS RELATED TO STRESS AFTER ITS OCCURRENCE— PTSD

The focus turns to what institutions can make in terms of prevention beyond a careful personnel selection. A lot of attention has been given to preventive activities at times of crises, disasters or incidents, particularly regarding Post-Traumatic Stress Disorder (PTSD. According to the DSM-IV, the criteria required for the diagnosis are:

- the existence of a clearly recognizable traumatic event such as an assault to the physical integrity, either of the individual or of a third party, which has been experienced either directly or indirectly by the affected person and which causes them fear, distress, or horror
- the repeated reexperiencing of the event (recurrent and intrusive thoughts, flashbacks, nightmares, and behavior as if the event was happening again)
- affective insensitivity (identifiable by a significant decrease in the interest in performing ordinary or significant activities, particularly if it has some relation with the traumatic event); feeling of alienation in relation to other people; affective restriction; inability to love
- psychomotor activation (hyperactivity, sleep disorders, difficulty concentrating, irritability)

Evidence shows that among police officers those who are more vulnerable to experiencing PTSD symptoms are those who have a family history of psychiatric disorders and substance abuse (Inslicht et al., 2010). However, we must take into account, in addition to individual variables, the organizational environment that may work as a buffer or mediate the relationship between exposure to critical events and the development of PTSD, related both to work activities and the personal life (Maguen et al., 2009). Generally speaking, organizational stressors have a strong effect, including the exacerbation of PTSD symptoms, which highlights the importance of continuously considering these issues because public security workers are being constantly exposed to situations that potentially could lead to the development of this disorder.

However, the predictor of highest risk for PTSD is peritraumatic dissociation, which refers to dissociation, in traumatized individuals, between the self who observes and the self who experiences (Kolk, McFarlane, & Weisaeth, 1996). People report they mentally leave their body at the time of the trauma and observe it happening from far. This process lessens pain at the time and protects against the total impact of the event. Dissociation can take the form of a feeling of time unchanged; either too slow or too fast, or still depersonalization, out-of-body experiences, bewilderment, confusion, disorientation, altered perception of pain, altered perception of one's own body, tunnel vision, and immediate dissociative experiences (Maia, Moreira, & Fernandes, 2009). This mechanism can be adaptive during the traumatic event; however, its subsequent use for coping with feelings when recalling the episode can lead the individual to a failure in the processing of the trauma and the meaning and emotions connected to it. Occasionally it may result in the development of even more severe symptoms, like the ones found among Canadian police officers by Marin and coworkers (Marin, Marchand, Boyer, & Martin, 2009).

After the September 11 attack to the World Trade Center in New York, several researchers conducted studies targeting professionals and volunteers who worked in rescue teams. It is interesting to notice that the prevalence of PTSD among volunteers is three times greater than among police officers. The hypothesis proposed to explain this result, in the case of the U.S., is the previous training to cope with emergency situations and the previous exposure to events of this nature.

Regarding previous training, American researchers recommend that public security agencies adopt the *Critical Incident Stress Management-CISM* (Mitchell & Everly, 1996) model. The model is designed to decrease the impact and strain caused by the event, facilitate the normal recovery process in regular people who have regular reactions to abnormal events and the recovery of the adaptive function. The principles of intervention include:

- Simplicity—people respond to what is simple, not to what is complex when they are facing a crisis
- Brevity—it should last minutes, at most one hour, in 3 to 5 sessions
- Innovation—it should use creativity to deal with new situations
- Pragmatism—suggestions should be practical
- Proximity—the most effective contacts or interventions are those made closest to the individual
- Immediacy—the crisis demands quick intervention
- Expectation—the person providing the intervention should work to raise expectations of a positive result.

CISM consists of seven components, which are the following:

1. Pre-crisis preparation—training to deal with and resist stress and overcome the crisis
2. Support programs for disasters or serious incidents at schools or communities, including mobilization, informal briefings, meetings, and staff counseling
3. Defusing. Discussion in a small structured group, in three phases, a few hours after the event, with the purpose of identifying, screening and minimizing acute symptoms
4. Critical Incident Stress Debriefing (CISD), which refers to a structured group discussion that usually takes place one to seven days following the event, designed to minimize and suppress acute symptoms, checking follow-up needs and, if possible, give people the feeling of closure regarding the issue
5. Individual psychological counseling, follow-up or support during the crisis
6. Intervention at the organization
7. Subsequent follow-up and additional treatments, if required

It is important to clarify here that the model described above is not psychotherapy, but rather an immediate response or "first aid" for the situation. There are many interventions that can be used to control the effects of crisis. However, even researchers who stress the effectiveness of the model or even the use of the debriefing strategy alone warn that the team leading the process should be properly trained. When properly conducted, debriefing represents closure: comparing it to a funeral, it is a ritual that gives people a closure; however, when the deceased is someone very close to the individual, the funeral is just the beginning. Therefore, debriefing is just the beginning for those who have been highly impacted by the event. Still, it can effectively work for most of those involved.

Although the CISM model shows up often in Canadian and American research studies on public security and social defense workers, it should be noted that its application in Brazil should be preceded by extensive research to check if it could possibly be applied to our culture and if it would be valid here. It is just one alternative to be used when facing PTSD and other psychological disorders or sources of stress. Additionally, it is one of the actions related to the promotion of quality of life, which is a broad and comprehensive concept involving healthcare, education, culture, social and family, leisure, social economic, affective and emotional status.

REASONS TO IMPLEMENT QUALITY OF LIFE AND STRESS REDUCTION PROGRAMS

At a time when resources are limited and with so many other urgent needs, people frequently question why specific programs should be implemented for these workers. The United States Department of Justice (available at http://www.ojp.usdoj.gov/nij/pubs-sum/163175.htm) outlines some reasons: providing a confidential and specialized approach to treatment and stress reduction for law enforcement officers and their families, improving their ability to cope with stress themselves, since they resist looking for external help; lifting morale and productivity; increasing the efficiency and productivity of the public service offered; decreasing the number of early retirements related to disabilities caused by stress; reducing the number of occupational accidents; reducing the number of lawsuits related to inappropriate behavior by law enforcement officers; reducing the negative attention by the media; and improving the overall well-being of police officers. Additionally, the document mentions the cost-benefit of the financial investment made in programs that prevent early retirements and unnecessary expenditures with healthcare or lawsuits.

However, in addition to all these features, biopsychosocial care provided to these workers means that the state is supporting those who chose to be constantly at risk in the exercise of their duty. Furthermore, it means taking care of the quality of life and the human rights of these officers so that they too can provide quality of life and respect the human rights of community members, acting as true transformers of society and protectors of citizens.

However, in order for concrete progress to be achieved in this area, agencies have to stop just providing care and start implementing activities and taking actions geared almost exclusively towards alleviating stress symptoms and working on prevention, establishing permanent people management policies that place law enforcement officers at the center of their issues; those policies should adapt the work to workers in order to achieve greater efficiency, effectiveness, better performance, better quality of life and, as result, impact the services provided to society. We have to reconsider this model of care in which a psychologist heroically tries to deal with the conflicts faced by a whole group of law enforcement officers, while the causing factor continues to exist. Additionally, strategies should be adopted at the individual and organizational level, including the officers' families, which can be a considerable source of stress or a source of support. Additionally, the families of the officers themselves may face difficulties or feel threatened by the work of their spouse or parent. In fact, in law enforcement care and prevention should coexist, since the risk factor will always be present. Even if management is changed, regulations reviewed and work conditions and hours are improved, dealing with the worst society has and with human drama will always be part of the work of law enforcement officers. We still have a long way to go until all goals set by the Quality of Life Project and set forth by Normative Guideline GAB MJ 01/10 are achieved. The diversity of cultural, structural, and social characteristics of every agency, of every community where they operate means that we must have specific and local plans. However, recognizing the predictors and protective factors, as well as the mechanisms to cope with stress, can help design more effective programs for the promotion of quality of life and health for law enforcement officers who put their own lives at risk every day when carrying out their duties due to the very nature of the law enforcement and social defense activity and the resulting exposure to constant extreme situations.

REFERENCES

Babin, B.J., & Boles, J.S. (1996). The effects of perceived co-worker involvement and supervisor support on service provider role stress, performance and job satisfaction. *Journal of Retailing, 72,* 57–75.

Department of Justice. (2010). Developing a law enforcement stress program for officers and their families. Retrieved from http://www.ojp.usdoj.gov/nij/pubs-sum/163175.htm

Dobreva-Martinova, T.D., Villeneuve, M., Strickland, L. & Matheson, K. (2002). Occupational role stress in the Canadian forces: Its association with individual and organizational well-being. *Canadian Journal of Behavioural Science, 34,* 111–121.

Ferreira, M.C., (2006). Qualidade de Vida no Trabalho (QVT). In A.D. Cattani, L. Holzmann (Eds.), *Dicionário de trabalho e tecnologia* (pp. 219–222). Porto Alegre, RS:Editora da UFRGS.

Glenn, R. W., Panitch, B. R., Barnes-Proby, D., Williams, E., Christian, J. Lewis, M. W., . . . Brannan, D. W. (2003). *Training the 21st century police officer: Redefining police professionalism for the Los Angeles Police Department.* Santa Monica, CA: Rand.

Hackett, R. D. (2002). Understanding and predicting work performance in the Canadian military. *Canadian Journal of Behavioural Science, 34,* 131–140.

Hughes, J. (2001). Occupational therapy in community mental health teams: A continuing dilemma? Role theory offers an explanation. *British Journal of Occupational Therapy, 64,* 34–40.

Inglehart, M. R. (1991). *Reactions to critical life events: A social psychological analysis* (1st ed.). Westport, CT: Praeger Publishers.

Inslicht, S.S., McCaslin, S.E., Metzler, T.J., Henn-Haase, C., Hart, S. L., Maguen, S., Neylan, T.C., & Marmar, C.R., (2010). Family psychiatric history, peritraumatic reactivity, and posttraumatic stress symptoms: a prospective study of police. *Journal of Psychiatric Research, 44*(1), 22–31.

IPEA. (2003). *Políticas sociais—Acompanhamento e análise, 7,* 90–95. Available at http://www.ipea.gov.br/portal/images/stories/PDFs/politicas_sociais/APRESENTACAO7.pdf

Jones, B., Flynn, D., & Kelloway, K. (1995). Perception of support from the organization in relation to work stress, satisfaction and commitment. In S. Sauter & Murphy (Eds.), *Organizational risk factors for job stress* (pp. 41–52). Washington, DC: American Psychological Association.

Kolk, B.V.D., McFarlane, A., & Weisaeth, (1996). *Traumatic stress: The effects of overwhelming experience on mind, body, and society.* New York, NY: Guilford.

Maguen, S., Metzler, T.J., McCaslin, S.E., Inslicht, S.S., Henn-Haase, C., Neylan, T.C., & Marmar, C.R. (2009). Routine work environment stress and PTSD symptoms in police officers. *Journal of Nervous and Mental Disease, 97*(10), 754–760.

Maia, A.C., Moreira, S.H., & Fernandes, E.E. (2009). Adaptação para a língua portuguesa do Questionário de Experiências Dissociativas Peritraumáticas (QEDP) numa amostra de bombeiros. *Revista de Psiquiatria Clínica, 36*(1), 1–9.

Marin, M., Marchand, A., Boyer, R., & Martin, N. (2009). Predictors of the development of posttraumatic stress disorder among police officers. *Journal of Trauma Dissociation, 10*(4), 451–468.

Mitchell, J.T., & Everly, G.S., (1996). *Critical incident stress debriefing: An operations manual.* Ellicott City, MD: Chevron.

Secretaria Nacional de Seguranca Publica—SENASP. (2006). *Relatório de Gestão.* Brasília.

Souza, E.R., & Minayo, M.C. (2005). Policial, risco como profissão: Morbimortalidade vinculada ao trabalho. *Ciência & Saúde Coletiva, 10*(4), 917–925.

Stacciarini, J.M.R., & Tróccoli, B.T. (2000). Instrumento para mensurar o estresse ocupacional: inventário de estresse em enfermeiros (IEE). *Revista Latino-Americana de Enfermagem, 8*(6), 40–49.

Tetrick, L. (1992). Mediating effect of perceived role stress: A confirmatory analysis. In J. Quick, L. Murphy, & J. Hurrell, Jr. (Eds.), *Stress and well-being at work* (pp. 134–152). Washington, DC: American Psychological Association.

Vasconcelos, T.S., (2005). *O Inventário Fatorial dos Cinco Fatores de Personalidade no Ambiente de Trabalho.* 2005. 159 f. Tese de Doutorado. Universidade de Brasília, UnB. Brasília, DF.

Wang, Z., Inslicht, S.S., Metzler, T.J., Henn-Haase, C., McCaslin, S.E., Tong, H., Neylan, T.C., & Marmar, C.R. (2010). A prospective study of predictors of depression symptoms in police. *Psychiatry Research, 175*(3), 211–216.

CHAPTER 9

QUALITY OF LIFE AND BURNOUT IN PHYSICIANS

Avelino Luiz Rodrigues, Elisa Maria Parahyba Campos, and Guilherme Borges Valente

First of all, we should try to establish the meaning of *quality of life*, which is not very easy since it is an extremely vague term. This concept provides us with broad definitions involving different categories of life, and makes it difficult to reach a consensus on this topic (Bernal, 2010). According to Assumpção et al. (2000), quality of life is a global concept approaching different facets in the life of an individual, such as health, family and environment, covering a variety of concepts ranging from physical conditions to social performance, including subjective ideas about well-being and satisfactory participation in a cultural context.

Bernal (2010) refers to the definition proposed by the Quality of Life Group of the World Health Organization: "an individual's perception of his position in life, in the context of the culture and systems of values in which he lives, and regarding his goals, standards and concerns" (p. 20). According to Forattini (1996), "Quality of life concerns the human condition and one might consider it as satisfaction with life" (p. 332); others define it as "satisfying basic needs that ensure a given standard of living of a person, family or population" (Kayano, 1996, p. 344); later "the subjective compo-

Coping and Prevention, pages 147–172

nent of the notion of well-being and happiness" (Barros, 1996, p. 344) was added to the concept. Likewise, two other terms that are not only adjacent to it, but also constituents of the meaning that we usually connect to quality of life, should be spelled out: *living condition* and *lifestyle*.

Living condition is understood as the way of living, resulting from social and economic class, thus including socioeconomic and demographic data. Lifestyle is the personal trait, the way of acting, of behaving and dealing with different situations of life, including people, and types of behavior.

A person's quality of life consequently includes living condition and lifestyle. Thus we can point out that a person has a good quality of life insofar as they have a good home with electricity, basic sanitation, access to effective health and education services, appropriate working conditions that will guarantee that they have a level of income ensuring healthy nutrition, opportunities for leisure inside and outside the home, and a healthy and efficient way of behaving towards life and its challenges. Additionally, quality of life includes a way of dealing with distress, including that resulting from work, creatively and constructively, without prejudices or emotions such as envy, jealousy, or competition, and the possibility of participating in groups and communities. But the notion of quality of life goes further; it is also related to a range of qualitative and quantitative characteristics of a person, and these may determine their well-being and safety. Limongi França (1994) reminds us that "people's expectations and cyclic needs for affection, economic issues, pattern of consumption, influence of peers or groups with whom the person lives, often unconsciously determine the indicators of quality of life which are important and valued for each person or group, at different moments" (p. 1).

In the aspects of quality of life more strongly influenced by a range of qualitative and quantitative characteristics, we easily perceive that they vary greatly from person to person. *Living well and pleasurably* (Limongi França, 1994), one of the definitions of quality of life, is not a homogeneous notion or idea in society, nor even in a segment that has a rather specific culture such as the medical community. If we were to perform a survey about what is considered quality of life in this well delimited segment of society, we would get many different answers. Some would focus their answers on living condition, others on lifestyle, and some on a mixture of both of these.

It is worth mentioning that the topic of quality of life has received growing attention in medicine. The International Health-related Quality of Life Society (Barros, 1996) was founded in 1964. The Medline system had 1,484 articles in 1993, 1,360 in 1994, and 1,596 in 1995. In a recent internet search, this topic has 93,687 citations. In a current Google search for *scholar*, 641,000 references to the term quality of life have been found.

This movement of medical sciences is seen as a "development of knowledge and of the complex social progress of the current times, which no longer allows understanding the health–disease process in its biological dimension alone, disconnected from the determinants associated with human relations" (Junqueira, 1996, p. 344). This reference, picked up by public health researchers, expresses the ideal underlying the establishment of the Associations of Psychosomatic Medicine at the end of the 1930s, at the international level, and in the 1960s in Brazil.

When the Brazilian Association of Psychosomatic Medicine was founded in 1965, the promotion of health began to be markedly defined within the boundaries of biopsychosocial principles (ABMP, 2011). Brazilian psychosomatic medicine began to include the processes of falling ill not as a casual event in a person's life, but as a response of an individual who lives in society, in constant interaction with other people, who is an active element in a family microstructure, part of the social and cultural macrostructure, situated in a given physical environment, and who seeks to solve his existence in the world as best as possible (Rodrigues, Campos, & Pardini, 2010). That is why quality of life is important if we are to understand human beings, insofar as it covers different aspects of life in an organism that is constantly interacting with the internal and external environment.

The vast majority of medical research involving the topic of quality of life tries to find out what are the effects of a given treatment on the impact certain diseases have on the patient's quality of life. Much more recently some researchers turned their attention to the quality of life of physicians. We think that this move should be seen as part of the "healthcare crisis, in the context of the social crisis marked by exclusion, inequity and violence, interpreted by many as unavoidable and even natural" (Kayano, 1996), which victimizes patients and physicians alike.

An editorial in the *British Medical Journal*, signed by the editor, Richard Smith (2001), refers to a feeling of relative unhappiness observed among physicians. The conclusion is that all physicians feel unhappy. This feeling is not seen all the time, but when physicians get together, their conversations are mainly about the problems and anxieties of their working conditions. The editor points out that the British government is concerned about this unhappiness among physicians, and acknowledges that a health service with demoralized physicians cannot prosper. He concludes: "The most obvious cause of physicians' unhappiness is that they feel overworked and undersupported."

Suspicions about an effective health care system and the excessive workload of medical professionals are no different in Brazil, as attested by the Federal Council of Medicine: "The lack of actions to respond to the issues worries us and leave Brazilians without the prospects for a future in health care" (D'Ávila, 2010). From the same perspective, a survey showed a significant apprehension among the population regarding the health care system (Jornal da Associacao Medica Brasileira, 2011a). The Federal Council of Medicine reveals that physicians, mostly, subject themselves to three or more activities, and the vast majority are pessimistic about the future of the profession (Carneiro & Gouveia, 2004).

Physicians seek to fulfill many expectations in the profession, "rewards" that we can classify as *internal* and *external*. The internal rewards are the physician's feeling that he is making people's lives better and that society should acknowledge and value his efforts. Often these internal rewards are not being given, which leads to intense feelings of frustration and disappointment with the profession. Many physicians, then, search intensively for external rewards, such as increased earnings and unceasing acquisition of material things, deluding themselves that this will enhance their quality of life. However, it is clearly perceived that the feeling of *something missing* persists.

In medical circles, however, this type of reward is not given, or only very rarely, be it because the State does not compensate physicians in a fair manner, or because the medical space is almost completely dominated by financial corporations—health insurance companies, private cooperatives, group medicine. Health has become just another item for sale. And in this game of power, for which physicians were not and are not trained, they are suffering an overwhelming defeat. There are fewer opportunities for external reward, insofar as, since the physician is also an item on sale, cheap and plentiful, because there are more than 200 thousand physicians competing at the labor market, the logic of the system itself has lead to the lower salaries.

The survey Perfil dos Médicos no Brasil (Profile of Physicians in Brazil) (Machado, 1997) revealed that the monthly income of a Brazilian physician was around US$1,163 in the capital cities and US$1,600 in the interior. Currently the minimum salary of physicians is three minimum wages, or around US$745 (JAMB, 2011a). In a more recent survey performed by the Federal Council of Medicine (Carneiro & Gouveia, 2004) a monthly income is shown as predominantly up to US$2,000, 72% receiving less than US$3,000 and only 8.5 % earning above US$4,000. The result of this is that the vast majority of these professionals end up working in three or more jobs.

Physicians have reported that, in the last five years, when compared to the survey, their compensation did increase but it came with an increased work load in hours, technical competence requirements, and bureaucratization of their services when they have to work for health insurance companies. Also, concerning the profession, the survey shows that most are satisfied with their specialty, but that the professional practice wears them out. As to the future, most are pessimistic and losing motivation because of the uncertainty in their profession. In fact, only 15% were optimistic.

The consequences of this set of circumstances on the quality of life of a vast majority of physicians are devastating. What we have today are worn out professionals (Rodrigues, 1998). Their living conditions are very far from those of which they dreamed. A study shows that almost all physicians

(92%) suffer some kind of interference with their technical autonomy by health insurance companies (JAMB, 2011b).

Considering all that has been said, together with a lifestyle that has been compromised, with little time for themselves and their families, many physicians are demoralized, constantly irritated, frustrated, socially isolated, and feeling that society does not acknowledge their work, with less social support and diminished idealism about the profession. There are signs of considerable levels of burnout (Rodrigues, 1998). A special edition of *BMJ Careers (Chambers, 2003)* dedicated to physicians' well-being *informs* "that excessive workload and absence of support are directly caused by poor working conditions."

Intrinsic aspects of the medical profession, such as long working hours, often with unforeseen events; involvement with major emotional aspects of the patients for which they were not trained, such as death, suffering, fear, sexuality; having to deal with the uncertainty of diagnosis and prognosis; and therapeutic possibilities that are not always very appropriate to the patients` needs, diagnostic tests that are not accurate, time pressure at work, inadequate training in psychology are factors that also compromise the physicians' quality of life, as powerfully as most organizational aspects that we mentioned previously (Rodrigues, 1998). And we will discuss them further on, in the nonspecific and specific sources of stress in medical practice.

Some indicators showing how physicians' quality of life is compromised are worth mentioning: In some countries, especially in Northern Europe, the medical profession is considered a risk factor for suicide. A study by Paykal, cited in Olkinuora et al. (1990) on thoughts of suicide among Finnish physicians showed the following:

- 11.5% of the physicians interviewed stated that at some point in time their life did not have meaning
- 8.2% that at some point in life they had a death wish
- 4.8% said that they thought about suicide
- 2.6% seriously considered suicide
- 1.1% attempted suicide

McCue (1982), in a classical paper on stress in physicians, says that the following evidence shows the high degree of stress medical professionals are subjected to:

- A suicide rate two to three times higher than the population in general
- A higher prevalence of alcoholism among physicians, compared to the population at large

- Thirty to one hundred times more frequent drug use than the rest of the population
- Tendency to use 1.6 times more "heavy drugs" than the control groups

In a survey of physicians who presented professional stress syndrome when they were subjected to situations of chronic stress, Singsen (1989) found the following data:

- 3% of physicians presented clinical manifestations of depression
- One third of them presented subclinical symptoms of depression

Frasquilho (2005) talks about medical work and its influence on the quality of life of these professionals.

- Physicians have more family conflicts and divorce twenty times more than the general population.
- They have a higher prevalence of anxiety, insomnia and depression than the general population.
- They have greater dependence on alcohol and drugs than the general population.
- Most of them neglect their own health, and do not have check-ups or do not see a physician.
- When some problem is diagnosed, generally they include several other diagnoses.
- Their rate of surgeries is three times higher than that of the general population.
- They demonstrate a low compliance with medical treatment, refusing, ignoring, or depreciating it.
- They deny or make light of the risks inherent in their professional practice.
- They minimize their personal indisposition.

SOURCES OF STRESS IN MEDICAL PRACTICE

There is a kind of conspiracy of silence around the topic of stress, to which physicians may be exposed in their daily medical practice. This can be found both in patients and in physicians, which is an obstacle to going further into the topic, although the review of literature shows a clear increase in the number of scientific papers published on this topic in the *Index Medicus* in recent years (Rodrigues, 1998).

Although physicians spend more than one third of their life preparing for their profession, which requires constant updating, they rarely recognize the psychological wear caused by this practice. They also find it difficult to recognize the conflict between their professional expectations and frustrations, and the requirements of reality in daily medical practice. For a long time, physicians or medical students believed that the pressure of the profession would be compensated by financial earnings and social status (McCue, 1982). Nowadays, however, this is not a certainty or even a reality. The jobs available may have very little to do with their vocation or their capacity to deal with emotional aspects or with patients of a social-economic-cultural level different from their own. At medical school future physicians are not prepared for the different situations inherent in the profession. Feelings and emotions are often suppressed in learning.

Unfortunately, medical schools do not teach students how to deal with their emotions. Indeed, emotions are not even supposed to appear in a medical visit. Physicians are taught that they should keep a certain distance from the patient, since emotional involvement may impair their professional performance. And, worst of all, most really believe this fallacy. Honest discussions about psychological difficulties in medical practice, or how physicians behaved in medical visits that involved very difficult situations are very rare, unfortunately, since they would help physicians to identify inappropriate adaptations and would help them learn to deal with situations without suppressing feelings, avoiding an excessive emotional distance that tends to compromise the development of an appropriate doctor–patient relationship. In general, these aspects are treated as secondary, where the problems in the relationship with the patient or the profession are covered up—or sometimes treated ironically—as though to suggest that the students or residents who have gotten involved in such difficulties are "weak" and "incapable." It is alleged that emotional "asepsis" is important to ensure self-control and maintain the technical quality of the intervention. In practice, what one gets are physicians who are not trained to deal with many truly stressful intrinsic aspects of the profession.

Fortunately efforts have been made to acknowledge the aspects mentioned above. The American Medical Association (AMA, 1979, cited in Nogueira Martins, 1998) showed concern about the physical wear and mental distress of resident physicians, and tackle this issue it set up a working group to develop models for the prevention and rehabilitation of these physicians. The result of this work was a book entitled *Beyond Survival — The Challenge of the Impaired Student and Resident Physician* (Tokarz, Bremerr, & Peters, 1979). Among the recommendations made in this book, it proposed (1) emphasizing the importance and severity of the problem of physical wear and mental distress (physician impairment) not only among residents, but among all physicians and (2) stimulating all residents to recognize the importance of preventing physician impairment during training and throughout medical practice.

It should be pointed out that learning to be a doctor is not a task that is done only with the force of motivation. The environment and social context where this learning takes place is very important; Delvaux, Ravazi, and Farvaques (1988) believe that depending on this environment, the student can construct adaptation strategies that favor a reduction or expansion of stressor impacts. Prior information about how internship would be helps adapt to this period of education. The author emphasizes that teaching at university should focus also on the psychological dimension of caring for patients; he criticizes medical training, saying that it is excessively directed at technical aspects, giving little or no attention to the problems inherent in the relationship between the professional and the person who is suffering and may die.

Nogueira Martins (1998) says that both the residents and the coordinators of medical residency programs should consider the different types of stress that should be carefully evaluated and considered in planning and organizing these programs. He also recommends the inclusion of psychopedagogical support of the residents. Such measures improve both the quality of professional training and the development of resources to deal with the stress inherent in training, as well as contributing to the quality of personal life. If, on the one hand the practice of medicine is often a source of much satisfaction, on the other hand there has been a great increase in dissatisfaction and suffering in the professional practice of medicine (Singsen, 1989).

Stress is intrinsic to the practice of medicine due to the very characteristics of the profession. It should be noted that often the same factor that can lead to gratification, fulfillment, and improved quality of work can also potentially cause symptoms that are usually described as resulting from the so-called burnout syndrome.

According to studies by McCue (1982), the main intrinsic stressors of medical practice are the following situations, considered specific to the professional practice of medicine.

MEDICAL WORK AND EMOTIONALLY CHARGED SITUATIONS

Suffering

The social encounters that make human interactions pleasant are much impaired by the presence of illness and pain. This frequently distresses people who suffer from them, making them unpleasant and often unable to show affection. When a physician deals with pain, he feels pressurized by the demands of the patient and the people with him. He has a medical training that makes him believe that a human being as a biopsychosocial being does not exist, and he is also not warned that he must control and supervise his own behavior. He was not warned that in the medical profession one receives very little compared to what is demanded. Besides, all the recognition, evaluation, and treatment of a patient in pain is based on the undeniable principle that someone else's pain is felt in a particular way by the physician; *the measure of the patient's pain can only be evaluated by the quantum of annoyance that is mobilized in the physician* (Schavelson, 1988). Contact with the patient's suffering constantly mobilizes annoying emotions that are, besides anything else, associated with elements of the physician himself, conscious and unconscious. The use of rationalization often assures the professional that the management was correct and that the best was done for the patient, but the unconscious does not always agree and this may cause suffering. Thus, other mechanisms may be triggered, but even so, another person's pain is only recognized if it provokes a certain conscious annoyance in the professional who treats the patient. This mobilizes very complex mechanisms.

Pain relief is entrusted to the physicians, but also the power of causing it, with certain medical interventions that have multiplied with the expansion of technology, providing an opportunity for more accurate diagnosis. It should be mentioned that no matter how modern and extraordinary the equipment, it only can yield better results in a direct proportion to the hand that operates it. A conflicted professional, frustrated in his work or ambitions and with financial problems, will not be very productive in his medical work, no matter what equipment he operates.

Fear

Pain is generally the definitive reason for the patient to decide to see a physician. However, often because of fear, patients postpone their visit and use rationalization mechanisms, sometimes presenting apparently very concrete reasons, such as the need to travel, work, or other things to do. "Denial mechanisms may also come into play, i.e., patients deny or minimize their symptoms, because they really fear both their disease and the physician" (Pontes & Rodrigues, 1980). Often it is difficult to deal with the illness, to accept its existence and its consequences. The decision to see the physician, for all and any patient, includes a set of conscious and unconscious elements from his personal history. The patient's decision to see a physician deserves much respect, as well as all the reasons for not having done so before (Schavelson, 1988). It is known that cancer patients often avoid going to the doctor, even when there are clear signs of illness. "It's a human trait that is independent of intelligence, knowledge or level of education the people's need to avoid admitting that they have a disease and its consequences, and avoid a diagnosis." "Physicians themselves, for instance, are no better patients than other people, despite their professional knowledge. They are pften those who most delay going to the physician, or try to avoid tests" (Tähkä, 1988). The patient's emotional situation is always ambivalent, because even with relatively simple tasks such as checking blood pressure, the possibility that the patient may die is being investigated. A calm and relaxed patient is so rare that the physician might think that it is this that really should be investigated. Fear is a biologically appropriate response to the threat of danger or loss. If it happens within reasonable limits, it motivates doing something to eliminate or avoid danger. When this danger is represented by symptoms of illness, the expected action is to make an appointment to see the physician, but reality shows that this does not always happen, and the reason for this behavior is fear. Here another important factor of stress appears for physicians. Physicians must know techniques for the appropriate management of situations in which patients are very anxious as a result of their medical conditions. However, physicians frequently ignore these practices, since they were not adequately taught them, because they are usually not part of the medical school curriculum, or if they are, they are part of the major subjects. Thus, physicians are forced to carry out a task for which they were not adequately trained.

With this "gap" in their professional training, physicians live in a situation that comes close to the concept of "stress" developed by Lazarus (1984), an event in which the internal or environmental demands exceed the adaptive resources of an individual.

Sexuality

The Hippocratic Oath specifically mentions this aspect: *In every house where I come I will enter only for the good of my patients, keeping myself far from all intentional ill-doing and all seduction and especially from the pleasures of love with women or with men, be they free or slaves.*

In few professions is a relationship so subject to eroticization as in the doctor–patient relationship. The physician is allowed and even encouraged to penetrate areas of the body that are not exposed to other people. The privacy of interaction with the patient, the atmosphere and confidential nature of the information given by the patient, his nakedness, exceptionally intimate examinations, the feelings of helplessness and dependency, and the transference phenomena caused by the regression due to the illness are factors that can lead to the development of a relationship that is not governed by the characteristics and rules of a professional relationship. The patient usually has contradictory feelings about the physician's privileged position, and the physician in turn may be torn between the wish to respect the patient's modesty, protecting him from the anxiety resulting from his physical and emotional nakedness on the one hand and the professional obligations and responsibilities of obtaining objective, concrete, and adequate clinical information on the other. Embarrassment is never entirely absent when you take a medical history and carry out a physical examination. The attempt to escape this stressful situation, even partly, may lead to an incomplete assessment of the patient and feelings of discomfort in the physician, because he did not follow the guidelines required by his training and experience.

Death

It is ironic to see that physicians who struggle to keep their patients alive are sometimes doomed to failure (McCue, 1982). The death of a patient is acknowledged as the greatest stressor for all health care professionals (Delvaux et al., 1988). Very often, the patient's death is seen as a failure by the patient's family and, sometimes, even by the doctor himself. This is only one of the impacts to which the physician is subject in this situation. Most physicians often work in the presence of death, but its proximity and even familiarity does not remove the anxiety it causes. Terminal patients personify this unpleasant emotion and may evoke aversive behaviors. Often interaction with the patient becomes insincere or cold and distant. When the physician's experience and knowledge indicate that the patient has a very poor prognosis this becomes a very different situation. However, maybe most difficult for the physician who deals with terminal patients is to think how the patient feels when he knows that his death is near. And this can be perceived by the physician in many ways: as a reminder of the limits of his knowledge, of the insufficiency of his resources and of science itself, a fact that is often placed in a hidden corner of the mind, besides the awareness of the limited extent of his own life and the memory of losses of people close to him. He may also feel that he failed and blame himself for not doing enough for the patient; he may be worried about the disappointment and possible criticism by the patient's relatives. Working with cancer patients causes chronic and cumulative stress. These professionals perceive their work as an excess load that is often beyond their resources and threatens their well-being, frequently accompanied by feelings of helplessness or even loss of self-esteem (Lazarus, cited in Delvaux et al., 1988) with the consequent development of burnout. It compromises the quality of care and creates a distance from the patient. The following reasons are given:

> I) there is a conflict between the expectations of cure which were strongly promoted in academic training, and the care that can be given to these patients, care which is generally palliative. II) Professional education does not provide adequate training to deal and communicate with these patients; III) because of their state, these patients tend to express feelings that are not always very easy to deal with, as for instance, anger, fear and depression ; IV) the difficulty of professionals to deal with the cumulative impact of consecutive, frequent deaths.

"For these reasons, professionals tend to keep away from these patients, because otherwise they will have to deal with the stress resulting from these wearing situations." Be as it may, death shows physicians their limits as combatants; its presence makes them feel smaller compared to the unrealistic, idealized image of omnipotent professionals. But, at the same time, the patients` demands for help, support, hope, and protection grow, and these expectations increase the feelings of impotence among the physicians, and often feelings of irritation and antipathy emerge in the patient. On the other hand, technological innovations can extend the process of dying. Physicians are placed in the highly stressful situation of determining the "death" of a patient when they decide to discontinue medications and switch off the equipment (McCue, 1982).

INADEQUATE TRAINING

Often some patients are easily labeled as "importunate," "whining," "refusing help," and many other distinctly pejorative terms. These attitudes show anger, fear, and often despair. The medical model, strongly based on biology, has poor resources to deal with such patients.

Another type of situation that should be highlighted in this topic is the idealized demands of society that come into conflict with uncertainty, a feeling that accompanies the daily life of any conscientious doctor. Medical education can be considered a learning process to deal with the uncertainty and limits of science. Making major decisions based on often conflicting and incomplete data is routine in medical work. Medicine is a "probabilities game" because it is not an exact science. This stress of uncertainty induces physicians to oversimplify the pathophysiology of the patient when he tries to explain why he is in this state. The result of this dialogue of "different dialects" is a number of misunderstandings and lies. This is expected to diminish fear, but when this untruth is discovered it affects the trust in the professional relationship.

Some characteristics of the work have a potential for affecting the biopsychosocial balance of the individuals involved. As to the medical task, some organizational stressors may be involved in (1) content and type of work,

(2) work organization, (3) responsibility, (4) role conflicts and ambiguous roles, (5) social relationships and "organizational climate," (6) relationships with the patients, (7) professional maintenance and development, (8) shift work, and (9) violence-related work (Rodrigues, 1998).

THE BURNOUT SYNDROME (BS)

The burnout syndrome (BS) is very complex. It can be investigated at different levels of organization, be it at the individual or at the organizational level. And, of course, approaching each of those levels requires using specific models and terminologies (Rodrigues, 1998).

Freudenberger launched the term *burnout* in 1975, followed by Maslach in 1976. The work of these pioneers focused mainly on emotional exhaustion, fatigue, and frustration in professionals as a result of wear and tear from contact with people, or the non-fulfillment of individuals' expectations and projects regarding their profession. The concept was positively received in the beginning (Maslach, 1984). After some time, however, severe criticism arose, such as that it was simply a new presentation of old themes or only on depressive manifestations. In response to the objections regarding the existence of the syndrome itself (Millan, 2007), Rodrigues (1998), Rodrigues and Campos (2010) support the consistency of the burnout syndrome (BS) construct, although BS bears some similarity to the depression responses resulting from adjustment disorders after a situation of stress and should be considered a separate syndrome because it is distinctly work-related and is usually temporary (Kirwan & Armstrong,1995); besides, it also presents a specific group of symptoms that always appear together, showing evidence of a recognizable entity (Paine, 1984).

There is a certain similarity between the symptoms of BS and the syndrome of essential depression described by Pierre Marty; in this condition there is no manifestation of depressive symptoms, and the individual continues to perform his daily activities without the significant symptoms of depression described in the psychiatric depressive syndromes or self-accusation. However, the relationship with the professional and social environment is impaired, and these individuals' interpersonal relationships become cold, distant, and without much affective involvement. The result is that they do not obtain pleasure from them (Diaz-Gonzales & Rodrigo, 1994). Although burnout and depression are often associated, several studies have shown that they are conceptually different (Vieira et al, 2006); the "state of depression" in burnout is temporary and geared towards a specific situation in an individual's life (Freudenberger, 1987) and it affects only the professional area, whereas depression affects all areas of the person's life (Maslach et al., 2001). Summarizing the differences between the syndrome of depression and burnout, in the latter: (1) people appear more energetic and are better able to take pleasure in their activities; (2) they rarely lose weight, present psychomotor impairment, and entertain suicidal ideas; (3) guilt feelings, if any, are more realistic; (4) they ascribe their indecisiveness and lack of activity to fatigue; (5) insomnia is more often initial, not terminal.

Barbosa et al. (2007) did a study in which they show research on burnout which distinguishes it from stress, because the latter may be both positive (*eustress*) and negative (*distress*), while the former is eminently negative. It is also different from the chronic fatigue syndrome, since this may be related to any sphere of a person's life, while burnout involves work. Although they are different from these constructs, they are closely related, so that they can trigger their symptoms.

Burnout means wearing out or becoming exhausted due to an excessive effort to respond to constant demands for energy, strength, or resources. It is one of the most important consequences of professional stress. Maslach (1982) described the burnout syndrome as follows: emotional exhaustion, depersonalization, and reduced sense of professional accomplishment.

- Emotional exhaustion: When a professional perceives that he does not have sufficient psychological resources to take care of others and give of himself, he feels worn out and lacks energy.
- Depersonalization: Here it is used in the sociological sense, and corresponds to the development of negative, insensitive and dehumanized attitudes by the professional towards the patients and people with whom he works.
- Reduced sense of professional accomplishment: This leads to a negative self-assessment. Generally physicians do not receive adequate and realistic feedback about their work and behavior in professional terms.

The following are the most frequently mentioned physiological indicators of BS: headache, tachycardia, muscle tension, anorexia, and insomnia. Psychologically, symptoms are expressions of rejection of situations experienced; frequent daydreaming, use of food, and tendency to sleepiness as forms of defense when dealing with situations of constant frustration; tendency to prepare for the worst; adopting negative attitudes, feelings of depression, and sometimes even symptoms of depression, intense anger, and feelings of hopelessness (Delvaux et al., 1988; Keller, 1989; Singsen, 1989).

It was also clear that these professionals often find it difficult to perceive these conditions and tend to react skeptically when help or suggestions are offered, and sometimes behave the same way to the patients. Often they say that they are tired, upset, feel withdrawn or irritated and tend to blame other people and/or organizations for their state. (Singsen, 1989).

In a study performed at a public hospital in São Paulo (Magalhaes & Glina, 2006) it was found that 11% of the physicians had burnout syndrome. The cases are distributed as follows: anesthetists, surgeons, and pediatricians, 25%; orthopedists and clinicians, 12.5%. As to professional activity: 62.0% of them work in the emergency room and 37.5% in other hospital departments; 62.5% of them work more than 61 hours a week and 100% hold more than three jobs.

Around 80% of physicians have moderate to high emotional exhaustion and depersonalization rates; the low rates obtained in professional accomplishment possibly account for the low prevalence of the complete syndrome (11%). These data appear consistent with the study by Carneiro and Gouveia (2004)

Tucunduva et al. (2006), in a study to find out the incidence of burnout among Brazilian physicians specializing in oncology, according to Maslach inventory, concluded that these professionals are particularly predisposed to this syndrome. It was observed at moderate or severe levels in the three dimensions in 15.7% of the physicians; 55.8% had a moderate or several level of emotional exhaustion. For depersonalization this number was 96.1%, and for reduced sense of professional accomplishment, 23.4%.

A SURVEY OF BURNOUT IN PHYSICIANS IN THE CITY OF SÃO PAULO

Procedures and Overview

Considering the aims proposed, we adopted qualitative methods for the investigation and interpretation of the data collected in the field, especially in analyzing the statements. The population studied consisted of practicing physicians—that is, possibly healthy individuals. The study objectives were to look at *stress* and *burnout* caused by professional practice by investigating their meaning (Spink, 1997) and their impact on physicians. The following procedures were chosen: (1) questionnaire—data for identification, professional training and reference to professional status; and (2) statements about the following questions: "What does medicine mean to you? Your professional practice? And what consequences does it have on your life?"

The Sample

After obtaining the consent of the *Associação Paulista de Medicina* (São Paulo Association of Medicine), we sent questionnaires to 351 physicians chosen randomly from the register of the Data Processing Department at that institution. We recommended that the physicians chosen have between ten and fifteen years of professional experience. Each of them received an envelope through the mail, containing:

1. a signed letter introducing the researcher and brief information on the survey objectives—*without specifying the terms stress or burnout*
2. information on how to complete the questionnaires attached and the statement, besides a guarantee that the information would be kept confidential
3. an addressed and stamped envelope with the author's address to which the answers were to be sent.

We received sixty-four questionnaires, or 18.23% of the total sent.

Analysis of Statements

Introduction

An example of the use of qualitative instruments to analyze health in Brazil is the work of Spink (1994a); analysis of the construction of knowledge on health, by Schraiber (1993); the study of physicians' narratives by Pitta (1990); Nogueira Martins' thesis (1994) on stress in residents whose attempt at understanding includes apprehending the meanings of their experiences and their actions, and the study on methodology by Turato (2003) in the Clinical-Qualitative Survey.

Methodology

The statements, stimulating reflections among the professionals, provided information that, besides intellectual elaboration, conveyed affective experiences on the type and quality of relations with medicine as a modality of knowledge, as well as the possibilities of intervention and the repercussions of professional practice on their lives.

Statements were chosen as a data collection technique in accordance with several determinations, some of them practical. It is easy to administer, it can be brief and delimit the topic, and material can also be collected through the mail. In this way, the subject of the study– stress and burnout resulting from professional practice—is not revealed, and therefore it does not influence the subjects' reports. On the other hand, the approach favors an associative flow of ideas on the experience and the different ways in which the subjects perceive it.

The objective of limiting the sample to physicians who have ten to fifteen years of professional work was to enable considerations on more mature experience of the profession—at least that was our assumption. Besides, the random choice of subjects made it possible to think about the statements of physicians, speaking about their daily experiences in their professional practices, concrete experiences, an elaboration of their daily life, a point of view concerning the present moment of medical practice "which is not always recorded."

The set of statements by the subjects reconstitutes a social moment, represented by physicians, by the different forms of practicing medicine, and by the different ways of experiencing and interpreting it. They spell out both the diversity and what is shared in the professional practice of medicine.

The following questions were asked: (1) "What does medicine mean to you?" (2) "What does the professional practice of medicine mean to you?" and (3) "How does it influence your life?"

Our intention was to extract the existence of stress from the statements, whether it is experienced as distress or not, whether it could result in burnout as a result of the impacts mentioned above, through the meanings they ascribed to medicine and its professional practice, and how these meanings mediated the stress process.

Before any comparative study, we read each statement by itself in order to pick up *the relationship between the individual and his professional practice.* The language used in the statements expresses a reflection on the experience and informs through its content not only by means of cognitive clarifications but also through the affective investment regarding the profession.

We used elements of the technique employed in the analysis of contents of interviews detailed by Spink (1994b). Based on this approach, the statements were divided into three groups:

- Group 1—There is no description of distress in the statement and the report is characterized by a satisfactory relationship with professional practice.
- Group 2—In the statement there is a report of a predominantly satisfactory relationship with the profession, but also the presence of distress in professional practice.
- Group 3—There is a report of distress in the statement and the discourse content is marked by a strong tendency to characterize an unsatisfactory relationship with professional practice and the presence of burnout.

Creating Categories

An attempt was made to map each discourse by asking the following questions: (1) Why does this subject feel that his professional practice is satisfactory? (2) Why does this subject feel that his professional practice is unsatisfactory? (3) What distress factors are present in the statement?

Obviously the first question was aimed at groups 1 and 2; the second question at Group 3, and the third question at groups 2 and 3. Next to each question we wrote the subject's answer. For instance:

A) Why is the professional practice felt to be satisfactory?

Subject 27: *"Medicine means my financial and psychological support, where I feel useful doing work that is significant for me and for the patients."*

Subject 35: *"I love to study and learn more about topics that interest me. . . ."*

B) Why is the professional practice felt to be unsatisfactory?

Subject 21: *"Medicine was and still is the greater ideal. However, much of the 'dream' is now over by far."*

Subject 56: *"If Hippocrates had lived in the days of the Brazilian Public Health System he would certainly never have worded the oath in this way."*

With this procedure we obtained a significant number of answers spelling out the reasons for a satisfactory or unsatisfactory relationship with the profession, and which factors of distress were perceived and reported.

Considering the variety of answers, namely the number of different perceptions about work, it was necessary to organize the descriptions in a way that would be appropriate to the objectives. We tried to group the answers according to categories that would represent them logically, that would apprehend common meanings present in the diversity of reports, categories that would spell out the meanings for the subjects, of professional practice based on practical knowledge (Sato, 1993), because they constitute activities reated to appropriate knowledge regarding experience acquired in this same pratice.

Thus, we built the categories using as a source of inspiration the very content of the subjects' discourse in the statements. They arose from the answers given to the questions. Namely, the categories that will be presented and will be used as a basis for the qualitative interpretation of the statements, although they can be considered integral parts of this process, did not exist until different answers were obtained to the questions asked. They arose as a movement proper to the scientific process, which is to try to organize a set of information that arose from the field data, to seek to apprehend and understand what is real.

RESULTS AND DISCUSSION

Demographic Data

Of the 64 physicians in the sample, 52 took a medical residency in a total of 21 specialties. Thirty-one physicians took a Specialization Course in a total of twenty-three specialties, and forty-nine subjects held the title of specialist.

Of the physicians who had the title of specialist, 34 work in their specialty and 29 subjects in other specialties. As to working with greater professional gratification, the outstanding choices are the office and teaching institution. The most often mentioned work places with the greatest possibility of professional advancement, were the office, private hospitals and teaching institutions. As to the weekly work load, 21 subjects work 40 hours or less, 15 work from 41–50 hours, 17 work 51–70 hours and 10 subjects work over 70 hours. Forty-eight of the subjects in the sample have offices; 23 of these subjects saw from 0% to 30% private patients, eight subjects from 40% to 90% private patients, and 17 subjects saw 100% private patients. The frequency of patients with medical insurance plans for 22 subjects is between 0% and 30% of the turnover in their offices; for 15 physicians it is from 40% to 90% and for five from 92% to 100%.

Presentation of Group Three

Report on distress and content of discourse with a strong tendency to show an unsatisfactory relationship with professional practice, with the presence of Burnout. According to the data collected, and comparing it to Group 1 in the sample, the subjects in Group 3 tend to be younger, a smaller number of them did medical residency or a specialization course, or they do not practice medicine in their respective specialty. Mostly, they do not practice at the places where they would get the greatest professional and financial gratification, a smaller number of them have the title of specialist, and they work longer hours. In Groups 1 and 2 there is no report of difficulties in acknowledgment of their work, lack of resources or proper conditions, or working with low income populations.

Categories Concerning Burnout

Pressure at work. Pressure for success, when dealing with the possibility of death and threats to the patient's well-being. These aspects, inherent in the medical work, are full of pain and suffering:

SUBJECT 07: *"(. . .) when something is going wrong it is stressful, tiring, urgent and difficult and you are alone (. . .) Medicine never deals with happy things, only with diseases, pains, troubles".*

SUBJECT 21: *" . . . "stress" is constant, because the cases that I usually see are very serious . . . ".*

Work overload. This is the fact that the profession requires that time be dedicated to it every day—including time for study—considered excessive:

SUBJECT 15: *"I work too hard, I study too much, and I participate in specialty meetings, courses, conventions, with no prospect of advancement, both professionally and in terms of quality of life".*

SUBJECT 54: *"Consequently, I have less time for my family and work more to be able to have a slightly better financial situation."*

Interference. There is interference from the professional activity in the personal and/or family life because of what is described above. Some reports, however, mention harmful interference in their personal life, not only as a result of excessive work, but also due to the degree of frustration and discomfort imposed by the profession.

SUBJECT 21: *" . . . working with a socio-culturally poor population, stress is constant because of the seriousness of the cases I usually see, and the great lack of resources available to me..(. . .) at the end of the day, the tension is so great , and also my doubts as to how useful I'm being (. . .) having lost a marriage because of my intense dedication to my profession ".*

SUBJECT 37: *"Medicine means everything, although it does not give me any financial and personal returns (. . .) I believe that I do not have much to grow (. . .) it is a career that* <u>*has lost much of its value*</u> *(underlined by the subject himself) in terms of fees; they do whatever they want to physicians (insurance companies, government, group medicine, etc . . .). A career where there is practically no place for praise, only for criticism. Although it is beautiful, I do not find any adjectives to describe the swamp in which medicine currently finds itself."*

The limits of intervention/of knowledge.

SUBJECT 21: *"there is constant stress due to the severity of cases I usually see . . . "*

SUBJECT 49: *"Medicine means science and the profession I chose to practice very early and without much information about the problems and limitations that I would encounter. In the specialty I chose (clinical oncology) I have a few moments of satisfaction and many of dissatisfaction, not only at the results obtained with current clinical approaches . . . "*

How the work is organized. Issues concerning how work is organized, relationship with colleagues, and lack of resources or conditions to do the work. Having to deal with low income populations, difficulty in entering the labor market, and institutional interference in medical work:

SUBJECT 07: "*. . . for the colleagues: a second-rate physician who keeps the patients quite when they operate. There is no acknowledgment, be it from the patient or from fellow physicians.*"

SUBJECT 15: "*Everything is very difficult, all the way from purchasing equipment, which is generally more expensive for the physician, to the professional practice itself, which is under a monopoly. A person graduates, goes to internship or residency, takes an exam to become a specialist, sets up an office and sees that he has no chance on the market. Then he goes looking for medical insurance companies, and comes home frustrated, because he is not a friend, or was not referred by someone to work for that particular insurance company. Insurance companies and group medicine organizations have a monopoly on the market. They took private patients out of the office and directed them to some professionals whom they have accredited.* "

SUBJECT 21: "*Currently, because I work at a poor municipal public hospital, in a low income neighborhood, with a socio-culturally poor population, there is constant stress due to the severity of cases I usually see and the lack of resources available to me. When it is not frustration about what you can prescribe, the patient goes to the pharmacy and chooses to buy one or two medications, not all those that were prescribed. Additional tests and hospitalizations are mostly prohibitive, and certainly, at the end of the day there is great tension, and also doubts about how useful I am being.*"

SUBJECT 24: "*Professional practice is very difficult, with a lot of competition, little incentive, and many colleagues wanting to see you fail . . .*"

Changes in the profession. The changes the profession has undergone in the subjects' imagination, the frustration of expectations that did not work out and the difficulties in having one's work acknowledged:

SUBJECT 07: "*Medicine, to me, meant (when I began to study): helping others, having a lot of knowledge and culture, participating in an upper social and financial class, overcoming challenges (. . .) There is no acknowledgment, be it by the patient or by colleagues.(. . .)*"

SUBJECT 15: "*Medicine was the greatest investment I made in time out of my life. I believed in the profession, but it did not bring me the desired professional and financial returns.*"

SUBJECT 54: "*Medicine, to me, would be the fulfillment of a great childhood dream, where I could practice a professional helping people and also feeling financially rewarded. (. . .) In practice, what we see is a total failure of the health care system, and a huge moral crisis in the people that run it . . .* "

CONCLUSION

The fact that, in the analysis of the statements, the answers were grouped into categories, apprehending common meanings present in the variety of reports, enabled us to reach a reality which is collective and shared by people in the group that comprises the sample.

The physicians in group three, in which the highest levels of burnout appeared, were the ones who had more issues regarding their professional accomplishment because of: A) the new forms of organization of the health care system, in the private system, characterized by the almost complete dominance of the institutions for which health is a market to be conquered; B) the precariousness of the conditions of professional practice, especially in the public health and group medicine services. Thus, these issues appear to expose physicians even further to the stress factors inherent in the profession, with more painful interferences in their personal and family life.

Another aspect, however, must be highlighted: these professionals are living in everyday situations of dissatisfaction, annoyance and distress in their professional lives, marked by the presence of a feeling of hopelessness in which the relationship with work is experienced as violence.

In order to better understand this aspect we refer to the notion of violence developed by Costa (1986), for whom it is an event derived from breaking a contract that had so far been implicit in the social order, a contract which expresses ideas that used to be shared and clearly present when the choice and training for this profession took place; the people—who suffered the action—shared those ideas and they were part of their identities, thus part of the way they saw the world and themselves. Furthermore, this breach of contract was arbitrary, using force, even though the agents of violence cannot be personified in a single subject, and can only be called State or market groups. *This breach of the social contract transformed several aspects of the relationship between these physicians and the professional practice into the emotional experience of violence, which can be seen in several reports, such as those of subjects, 7,15,21,54.*

The opportunities for a great majority of physicians to achieve the aspirations that were legitimized by the culture are removed during the course of their professional development. But they are not and cannot be easily set aside. A large investment was made in the profession and in training—both affectively and in financial terms and in time; possibly because of this the adherence of physicians to the profession is usually one of the greatest compared to the other professions, as emphasized by Machado (2001). Besides, from a certain top level of urban socialization, of competition for status, this aspiration is irreversible.

Some subjects in the sample try to continue the profession, defending themselves from this attack on the self, with expectations of future changes.

In others this no longer occurs. And, as we pointed out earlier, the relationship with the profession is marked by annoyance and distress, in a situation seen as having not way out, with no alternatives, and they tend to respond through pain-sparing psychological mechanisms.

We will develop this reasoning, because it allows us to understand how the mental representation of violence acts to determine the behavior of these people, insofar as important parts of the self, integrating the psychological type consistent with the identity built in the interrelationship with the social pattern of the group, are frankly under threat of destruction.

The experience of satisfaction is the main factor of growth and psychological development. Thus, when a person seeks situations of pleasure in reality, besides the aspects connected with satisfaction, they perform a movement that favors their personal development and helps them deal with the other situations that generated disappointment and annoyance. The thinking, by pleasure-displeasure polarization, go through the sphere of representations and affects that concern the pleasure of thinking and the possibility of experiencing pleasure again (Costa, 1986). In other words, of something that may be incorporated by the self. (Szasz, 1975). In the experience of pain, something different happens; it is associated with death and destruction, and to defend itself the psyche triggers defenses in order to control the painful experience, to make it disappear. There is a narcissistic reflux towards the Ego, with the development of stereotyped, mechanical, rigid, behaviors and actions that are an attempt at a more or less lasting affective neutralization of the experience.

These are ways of dealing with the violence by which the subject feels victimized. A violence that came from breaching a contract that was implicit in the social order and that legitimized the aspirations that sustain the very choice of profession. An arbitrary breach of contract, imposed and generating distress, felt as not having an alternative and threatening the subject's identity.

In Brazil, from the 1980s onwards, changes in the health care system were outlined, with two alternative modes of organization: the State owned one, now represented by SUS (Single Health System), and by the health care services of municipalities and states; and the other, private and business-centered. Thus, the autonomous and individual practice of medicine, considered a model of professional practice, slowly lost space.

According to Donnangelo (1975), these transformations can only be adequately interpreted based on processes that were concretely developed inside these societies and that transcend the sphere of medical practice, and are related to the transformations of an essentially urban and industrial society.

These aspects led to other changes in medical practice. The use of technology grew at a fast rate and became practically a standard of competence and efficiency. This led physicians to semiological and therapeutic practices based almost exclusively on technology, with less personal involvement. The survey: "Physicians in Brasl: a portrait of reality" confirms this statement (Machado, 1997).

According to the participants in this study, the medical practice, as it is being mediated by the State bureaucracy or by private companies, the resulting drop in remuneration, together with the demands for high productivity, excess work, technology prevailing over clinical knowledge, seriously compromise the relationship between physicians and the practice of their profession. All of this causes the *emotional experience of violence and the development of burnout.*

REFERENCES

Associação Brasileira de Medicina Psicossomática–ABMP (n.d.). *Estatuto.* Retrieved January 28, 2011, from http://www.psicossomatica.org.br//psicossomatica/default.asp?cod=44

Assumpção, Jr., F. B., et al. (2000). Escala de avaliação de qualidade de vida (autoquestionnaire qualitè de vie enfant imagè): Validade e confiabilidade de uma escala para qualidade de vida em crianças de 04 a 12 anos. *Arquivos de neuropsiquiatria, 58*(1), 119–127.

Barbosa, G. A., Andrade, E. O., Carneiro, M. B., & Gouveia, V. V. (2007). *A saúde dos médicos no Brasil.* Brasília: Conselho Federal de Medicina.

Barros, M. B. A. (1996). Qualidade de vida e saúde: Considerações de uma perspectiva epidemológica. *Reunião Anual da SBPC, 48,* 334. São Paulo, SP.

Bernal, M. P. (2010). *Qualidade de vida e autismo de alto funcionamento: percepção da criança, família e educador.* Dissertação de mestrado, (p. 20), Instituto de Psicologia, Universidade de São Paulo, São Paulo.

Carneiro, M.B., & Gouveia, V.V. (2004). *O médico e o seu trabalho.* Brasília, Brasil: Conselho Federal de Medicina.

Chambers, R. (Ed.). (2003). Physicians' well-being [Special Issue]. *British Medical Journal, 326.*

Costa, J.F. (1986). *Violência e psicanálise* (2nd ed.). Rio de Janeiro, Brasil: Edições Graal.

D'Avila, R.L. (2010). Editorial. *Jornal do Conselho Federal de Medicina, 25*(188), 2.

Delvaux, N., Razavi, D., Farvaques, C. (1988). Cancer care: A stress for health professionals. *Soc. Sci. Med., 27,* 159–166.

Diaz-Gonzales, R. J., & Rodrigo, I. H. (1994). El sindrome de "burnout" em los medicos del sistema sanitário público de salud. *Rev Clin. Esp. 194*(9), Madri.

Donnangelo, M.C. (1975). *Medicina e sociedade.* São Paulo, Brasil: Pioneira.

Forattini, O. P. (1996). A Sociedade Moderna e a Qualidade de Vida. *Reunião Anual da SBPC, 48,* 332. São Paulo, SP.

Frasquilho, M. A. (2005). Medicina, médicos e pessoas: Compreender o stresse para prevenir o burnout. *Acta Med Port, 18,* 433–444.

Freudenberger, H.J. (1975). The staff "burn-out" syndrome in alternative institutions. *Psychother Theory Res Pract , 12,* 73–82.

Freudenberger, H.J., & Richelson, G. (1987). *L'épuisement professional: La brûlure interne.* Otawa, Canada: Ed Gaëtan Morin.

Jornal da Associacao Medica Brasileira (JAMB). (2011a). Retrieved January 28, 2011, from http://www.amb.org.br/teste/imprensa/jamb/jamb_2010_jan_fev.pdf

Jornal da Associacao Medica Brasileira (JAMB). (2011b). Retrieved January 28, 2011, from http://www.amb.org.br/teste/imprensa/jamb/jamb_2010_mai_jun.pdf

Junqueira, V. (1996). Qualidade de vida e saúde e o SUS. *Reunião Anual da SBPC, 48,* 344. São Paulo, SP.

Kayano, J. (1996). Qualidade de vida e saúde. *Reuniao Anual da SBPC, 48,* 344. São Paulo, SP.

Keller, K.L. (1989). Management of stress and prevention of burnout in emergency physicians. *Annals of Emergency Medicine, 18,* 42–47.

Kirwan, M., & Armstrong, D. (1995). Investigation of "burnout" in a sample of British general practitioners. *British Journal General Practice, 45,* 259–260.

Lazarus, R.S., & Folkman, S. (1986). *Estrés y processos cognitivos.* trad. Maria Zaplana. Barcelona, Spain: Martínez Roca.

Limongi Franca, A.C. (1994). *Qualidade de vida—Da teoria à prática.* São Paulo: Insight.

Machado, M. H. (1997). *Os médicos no Brasil: um retrato da realidade.* Rio de Janeiro, Brasil: Editora Fiocruz.

Magalhaes, R.A.C & Glina, D.M.R. (2006). Prevalência de burnout em médicos de um hospital Público de São Paulo. *Saúde, Ética & Justiça, 11,* 29–35.

Marty, P. (1993) *A Psicossomática do Adulto.* p. 18. Porto Alegre : Artes Medicas Sul.

Maslach, C. (1976). Burned-out. *Human Behavior, 5,* 16–22.

Maslach, C. (1982). *Burnout: The cost of caring.* Englewood Cliffs, NJ: Prentice Hall.

Maslach, C. (1984). Understanding "burnout": Definitional issues in analyzing a complex phenomenon. In W. S. Paine (Ed.), *WS, job "stress" and "burnout": Research, theory, and intervention perspectives.* Thousand Oaks, CA: Sage.

Maslach, C., Schaufelli, W.B., & Leiter, M.P. (2001). Job Burnout. *Annual Rev Psychol, 52,* 397–422.

McCue, J.D. (1982). The effect of stress on physicians and their medical practice. *The New England Journal of Medicine, 306*(8), 458–436.

Millan, L. R. (2007). A Síndrome do Burnout: Realidade ou ficção ? Editorial. *Rev Assoc Med Bras; 53*(1), 5.

Nogueira-Martins, L.A. (1994). *Residência médica: Um estudo prospectivo sobre dificuldades na tarefa assistencial e fontes de "stress."* Doctoral dissertation, Universidade Federal de São Paulo—Escola Paulista de Medicina, São Paulo.

Nogueira-Martins, L. A., & Jorge, M. R., (1998). Natureza e magnitude do estresse na Residência Médica. *Revista da Associação Médica Brasileira, 44*(1), Mar.

Olkinuora M. et al. (1990). Stress symptoms, burnout and suicidal thoughts in Finnish physicians. *Soc. Psychiatry Epidemiol., 28,* 81–86.

Paine, W. S. (1984). *"Burnout" "stress" syndrome and the 1980s. Job "stress" and "burnout": Research, theory ,and intervention perspectives.* Thousand Oaks, CA.

Pereira de Sa, C. (1993). *Representações sociais: O conceito e o estado atual da teoria. O conhecimento do cotidiano: As representações sociais na perspectiva da psicologia social.* São Paulo, Brasil: Editora Brasiliense.

Pitta, A. (1998). *Hospital*–dor e morte como ofício. São Paulo: Editora HUCITEC.

Pontes, J. F., Rodrigues, A. L,. & Rodrigues, D. M. (1980). *Relação Médico-Paciente. Farmacologia.* Rio de Janeiro: Guanabara Koogan. p. 1252

Rodrigues, A. L. (1998). *Stress e Exercício Profissional da Medicina.* Doctoral dissertion. Faculdade de Psicologia, Pontífice Universidade Católica, São Paulo.

Rodrigues, A. L., & Campos, E. M. P. (2010). *Síndrome do Burnout. Psicossomática Hoje.* Porto Alegre: Artmed.

Rodrigues, A. L., Campos, E. M. P., & Pardini, F. (2010). *Mecanismo de formação dos sintomas. Introdução a psicossomática.* São Paulo, Brasil: Atheneu.

Sato, L. (1993). A representação social do trabalho penoso. In M.J.P. Spink (Ed.), *O conhecimento do cotidiano: As representações sociais na perspectiva da psicologia social.* São Paulo, Brasil: Editora Brasiliense.

Schraiber, L. B. (1993). *O médico e seu trabalho: Limites da liberdade.* São Paulo, Brasil: Editora HUCITEC.

Schraiber, L. B. (1995). Pesquisa qualitativa em saúde: reflexões metodológicas do relato oral e produção de narrativas em estudo sobre a profissão médica. *Rev. Saúde Pública, 29,* 63–74.

Schavelson, J. (1988). *Paciente com cancer.* Buenos Aires, Argentina: Cientifica Interamericana.

Singsen, B. H. (1989). Stress on the physician in practice. *Delaware Medical Journal, 61*(8), 401–406.

Smith, R. (2001). Editorial. *British Medical Journal, 322,* 1073.

Spink, M. J. P. (1994a). *A medicina e o poder de legitimação das construções sociais de igualdade e diferença: uma reflexão sobre cidadania e gênero. A cidadania em construção.* São Paulo, Brasil: Cortez Editora.

Spink, M. J. P. (1994b). *Desvendando as teorias implícitas: Uma metodologia de análise das representações sociais. Textos em representações sociais.* Petrópolis, Brasil: Vozes.

Spink, M. J. P. (1997). *O sentido da doença: contribuição dos métodos qualitativos em pesquisas sobre o câncer. A mulher e o câncer.* Campinas: Editorial Psy.

Szasz, T. S. (1975). *Dor e prazer: um estudo das sensações corpóreas.* Rio de Janeiro, Brasil: Zahar.

Tähkä, V. (1988). *O relacionamento médico-paciente.* Porto Alegre: Artes Médicas.

Tokarz, J.P., Bremerr, M., & Peters, K. (1979). *Beyond survival: The challenge of the impaired student and resident physician.* Chicago, IL: American Medical Association.

Tucunduva, L., Garcia, A., Prudente, F., Centofanti, G., Souza, C., Monteiro T., ... Gilgio, A. (2006). Incidence of the burnout syndrome among Brazilian cancer physicians. *Rev. Assoc. Med. Bras.,52*(2).

Turato, E.R. (2003). *Tratado de metodologia da pesquisa clínico-qualitativa: Construção teórico-epistemológica, discussão comparada e aplicação nas áreas da saúde e humanas.* Petrópolis, Brasil: Vozes.

Vieira, I., Ramos, A., Martins, D., Bucasio, E., Benevides-Pereira, A., Figueira, I., & Jardim, S. (2006). Burnout na clínica psiquiátrica: Relato de um caso. *Ver Psiquiatria, 28*(3), 352–356.

CHAPTER 10

HEALTHY POSSIBILITIES TO FACE A HYPERMODERN LIFE

Facets of Constructive Leisure

Ieda Rhoden

In this chapter I will discuss spare time and leisure from a psychological point of view and their relationship with health and quality of life, based on theoretical and empirical research on these subjects, among them my PhD research on Leisure and Human Potential, carried out at Deusto University (Rhoden, 2004). I would like to make clear now that although theoretically there are many conceptual differences regarding leisure experiences, I will focus more on the subjective dimension of these experiences, without wanting to go deeper into and distinguish these concepts.

My main goal is to discuss elements that are often forgotten or that do not get much attention in studies on leisure, namely the experiences of *rupture, rest,* and *introspective states* as healthy alternatives people can resort to in order to face hypermodern life styles and to recover their quality of life. When we use the term *experience* we refer to the phenomenon that is part of human existence that enables an individual to get out of him/herself and get in touch with reality, with other people, with objects, and ultimately with

Coping and Prevention, pages 173–192

the world. According to Boff (2002), experience results from the encounter with the world in a constant come-and-go that enables us to construct and also deconstruct mental representations generated by education or the society where we live. For this author, the encounter of the Self with the world is always enriching because it provides us with different ideas about reality. The knowledge resulting from this encounter is precisely what characterizes the "experience" we refer to. Knowledge coming from experience is verifiable knowledge. Being open and receptive, letting go of preconceived ideas are essential conditions for the experience. Experience, therefore, is the way we internalize reality and locate ourselves in the world and in relation to others.

Therefore, leisure experiences are healthy alternatives to fight stress and promote quality of life. However, these experiences must have certain characteristics experts call the psychosocial attributes or qualities of spare time and some leisure activities. Leisure experiences can occur as part of everyday activities or under extraordinary circumstances. Sometimes they manifest themselves as excellent states in which human capacities reach their peak (Csikszentmihalyi, 1997; Maslow, 1999), and at other times they occur as states of psychophysical recovery. Leisure can be experienced at different stages of life, by both genders, and by people from different social economic status and cultures. What separates the leisure experience from other types of human experience or even two or more leisure experiences from each other are the following factors: (1) the reasons that drive it and the psychosocial conditions under which it occurs; (2) the personal experience itself—that is, the thoughts, sensations, feelings, and emotions involved in the experience and their different levels of depth; and (3) the benefits resulting from the experience according to the perception of the individual.

Here we chose to adopt a systemic view and treat leisure as a psychosocial, dynamic, and procedural phenomenon that brings together all these characteristics. From a range of over 50 possible qualities or attributes that are part of leisure activities, some seem to be more widely accepted by authors, in addition to being theoretically more consistent and coherent in light of psychological science such as *the perception of freedom, intrinsic motivation or meaning; enjoyment,* and *sociability.*

Other attributes that are also identified as elements of leisure experiences seem to have relative theoretical importance, depending on the author and the specificity of the experience, such as the presence of *challenges,* the focus on the experience, the *aesthetic appreciation,* and the experience of *authenticity.* Nevertheless, in this chapter I would like to approach just some of the leisure attributes that are less valued or recognized by the specialized literature, but whose effects show their importance in the context of hypermodernity, particularly regarding health and quality of life. I refer to the phenomena of *rupture, rest, psychological involvement,* and *introspective states.*

In order to facilitate the understanding of these phenomena, we have grouped their qualities according to their psychodynamic interactions and their possible psychological effects on the individual having the experience. We will highlight here the following groups of qualities or attributes of leisure: distraction, evasion and rupture; rest and relaxation; the psychological involvement and concentration on the experience and finally, the introspective states: the encounter with oneself, with nature and with beauty.

From this point we will go deeper into what *rupture, rest* and *introspective states* mean taking as basic principles European theories of leisure and research in the area of Psychology of Leisure carried out in North America.

EVASION, DISTRACTION, AND RUPTURE

The attempt to find compensation, complement, or flight through distraction or entertainment guides behavior towards concrete actions that are characterized by changes of place, pace, and lifestyle or through fictitious activities supported by projections and resources of imagination. The search for entertainment in the attempt to break routines points to a strong relationship between contemporary leisure and the emerging demands of modern and post-modern urban life, such as getting away from everyday life, clearing the mind, evading problems, or simply getting out in the cathartic sense.

We are talking here about the necessary experience of getting away from and temporarily forgetting a specific situation that is connected to negative and unpleasant sensations and feelings. Therefore, distraction in this sense means the action of breaking away from a certain occupation or getting rid of some preoccupation. Parties and mass sports, as well as television are examples of activities that usually serve the purposes of distraction and evasion. However, every person must find his own form of distraction and evasion depending on what bothers him.

In some situations distraction can manifest itself as a difficulty in keeping attention or as a rupture of thinking resulting from excess stimuli that are so diverse that the individual is not able to pay attention to any of them. This means that distraction can result in a rather automated and unconscious behavior. An issue that is raised from this possibility is knowing if distraction or entertainment, as well as evasion and rupture, as described here, are able to bring benefits to individuals, in addition to the immediate and fleeting relief of some psychological discomfort.

What we know is that distraction may have two different connotations. On the one hand, it can be an experience of inattention, dazzlement, or even inadvertence when the individual is faced with various stimuli; on the other hand, it can be a relaxing experience—albeit a superficial one—that distracts and separates the individual from something that is a nuisance. We should recall that the very term *diversion*, proposed by Pascal (1979), indicates an occupation that prevents people from thinking about their essential issues. So, if we adopted a conception of diversion exclusively with this meaning—as something designed to prevent individuals from having to face and cope with human and existential issues—we would feel more comfortable in attributing to it the status of psychosocial symptom rather that of constructive leisure.

Gunter (cited in Tinsley, Tinsley, Hinson, & Holt, 1993) in his studies found that *separation from everyday life* and *fantasy* are characteristics of leisure and entertainment. Fantasy is the opportunity that leisure and entertainment can give us to experience or express an imaginary world, "another world." Considering these ideas we wonder what kind of society is this that urges us to live "in another way" and create "another world" in our free time and in leisure? Rather than giving an answer, we would like to prompt a reflection.

Rupture usually implies physical movement and/or psychological withdrawal that allows us to intentionally separate or temporarily forget a situation that is upsetting us, such as a tense work environment, professional or social pressures, concerns, or unpleasant feelings. Rupture can also present itself as the emphatic denial of doing and thinking or as the intentional choice of an activity that is totally opposite to what is known and habitual. For example, someone who is overstimulated at work could choose a leisure activity with extremely low levels of stimulation, while someone else who works in the absence of stimuli would choose a more exciting leisure activity. We understand that breaking with the monotony of routine, with inhibiting forces, with the external limitations of self-expression and with the sources of pain and distress is necessary and good for an individual's health and integrity, although this need may clash with the new forms of organization of modern and post-modern society.

Rupture strategies may vary, from an attempt to simply "not think at all," think only about things that do not require any effort, do something very different from what one is used to doing, change environment, life style or pace, let oneself be absorbed by different things or events, and so on. All these forms of rupture and distraction may coincide with personal constructive leisure experiences, provided they are different from states of personality dissociation, alienation and identity loss, in other words, of rupture from the Self. Therefore, the experiences of rupture promoted by any type of external agent will not necessarily match a concept of diversion in the humanist sense.

Finally, it is probable that the concrete need of flight or evasion, as well as of physical and mental rest has some influence on the choice of leisure and entertainment, making people prefer activities or situations that do not require efforts or significant chances, be it due to the mental representation of the activity or to what the activity really demands from the individual that carries it out. A fact that cannot be neglected is that the hypermodern society makes it easier and encourages individuals to frantically occupy themselves, even in their free time, often with consumerist activities that do not contribute to the establishment of a psychological and physical balance, let alone the improvement of their quality of life. This type of activity or occupation serves rather market interests and the social representations of belonging to a certain group or social class.

REST AND RELAXATION

Several research studies on leisure state that the experience of *relaxation* and *rest* constitute elements of the situations perceived and experienced as leisure. Dumazedir (1964) was one of the first theoreticians of leisure to affirm its resting function. According to this author, leisure protects individuals from wear and the physical or mental problems caused by the strains generated by obligations and routines.

Society has undergone important changes regarding life style in the past 50 years, particularly regarding communication systems, the organization of the market, of work and the family. This has made rest and relaxation factors that are increasingly important for human health. Modern life has significantly changed its natural cycle, increasing the speed of actions and thinking, at the expense of retreat, concentration and rest.

Saint-Arnaud (2002) suggests we should learn how to see the degree of tension that tires us, so that we could act preventively and maintain our biopsychosocial and spiritual balance. However, going against this recommendation, the fast pace of our lives limits our deep perception—that is, this pace tends to generate superficiality in our mental life and self-consciousness. With a more superficial level of consciousness, the quality of human perception is impaired and people cannot value abstract and subjective elements of reality, and values such as calm, serenity, and quality are either forgotten or they remain at the background. At the same time, contemporary society overvalues the material and quantitative dimension of reality, worshiping objects and images and quantifying data and facts. The psychoanalyst Maria Lucia Kehl stated in one of her lectures that we live in the realm of enjoyment (Kehl, 2003) that "we live in the realm of enjoyment—everything at the same time and now." Also for this psychoanalyst it is amazing that the seduction of the devices people use to adapt to the culture of narcissism and consumption still meets with resistance.

Maybe this is why, to compensate for a hyperactive day of work, individuals usually tend to surrender almost desperately to rest, diving into fantasies and illusory mechanisms to escape from reality. A clear example of this attempt is the fact that people turn the TV and the stereo on at the same time they do something else, like working on a computer or preparing a meal. In such situations, although the individual needs to rest, they can only get some distraction by replacing some stimuli with others, often maintaining an accelerated mental pace.

Although people have not been properly guided or educated as to how to properly rest, and although they often do not give enough attention to this task, they empirically try to find ways of decreasing their physical or mental activity, particularly in their free time. This is one of the reasons why rest, energy recovery, and relaxation can be considered qualities of leisure experiences.

From specific studies on the dynamics and effects of relaxation, we find that constructive leisure can contribute to this function with different levels of efficiency and depth. As mentioned previously, the simplest strategy in the search for rest is to replace one activity with another, which can generate a feeling of immediate relief without, however, resulting in actual rest—that is, without replenishing the energy and generating a psychophysical balance. It seems that leisure studies do not take into account these differences either, considering as relaxation and rest any experience perceived as such by those having it. However, we know that rest can have different qualities and significantly differ from deep relaxation.

In Fontcuberta (1976) we find a contribution about the psychophysical dynamics of movement and rest as a continuum. Life is made of two types of movement: contraction and dilation, and every human movement is the manifestation of these rhythms: centripetal movements that tend towards the inside, the center, and centrifugal, and expansive movements that tend towards the outside of the subject. These movements necessarily alternate with rest and relaxation. I contend that this applies both to the physical and the mental life.

Resting for people means to put into practice something different; to rest from attention they resort to imagination, to rest from external activities they resort to internal activities, and so on. Expanding this approach, we may say that there are three appropriate ways of resting: replacing an activity with another one, deep sleep, and conscious relaxation. These forms of resting may coincide or not with experiences of leisure, particularly the replacement of one type of activity with another and conscious relaxation.

The replacement of one activity with another is based on the alternate rhythm we have already talked about and is usually the means most people resort to in their attempt to rest, but it is also the least effective one because it leads to only partial rest and sometimes just causes a rupture from everyday life. The most common replacements, either conscious or unconscious, are classified as follows: replacement of a mental activity with a another activity of physical or emotional nature that will generate mental rest; replacement of an emotional-affective activity with a mental or physical activity generating rest of sensitivity; and the replacement of a physical activity with an activity of affective or mental nature that will make the body rest. In order for these strategies to work, the memories and images from the previous activity cannot mix with the new activity, which could result in a difficult task for some people.

Deep sleep depends on some conditions, such as good health, absence of affective and mental conflicts or unresolved issues—a possibility we think is rarely the case—and the sufficient use of the body and physical energy for several hours preceding the time of sleep. And finally, the third rest strategy is conscious relaxation which for some people may be a leisure experience in itself. It would be appropriate to better understand, beyond common sense, what the relaxation process is and how it works

Fontcuberta (1976) and Schultz (1969) explain that relaxation is the opposite of action, since every action presupposes a discharge of energy and relaxation is a way of replenishing this energy. Energy is spent at every muscle contraction; therefore the muscle contraction that does not have a purpose means energy loss, a rather common phenomenon today, when people contract their muscles as a response to an emotional strain or psychological repression. Certainly greater action or strain requires more relaxation and rest. The better the quality of the relaxation, the more energy will be accumulated, and the more energy an individual has, the greater will be his capacity to act.

From an organic point of view, relaxation means better blood flow, oxygenation, change in the respiratory level for a deeper breathing than usual, and smooth functioning of the cellular, muscle, digestive, metabolic and nervous system. Relaxation has the ability to slowly and safely relieve muscle strains, in addition to freeing us from mental hyperactivity, leading us to a state of calm and serenity. The relaxation experience generates well-being and if it is profound and systematic, it may cure physical and psychological conditions. According to Saint-Arnaud (2002), the pleasure of relaxation results from the integration and harmony between the physical and the spiritual and between oneself and others. Next we will have a chance to get to know other qualities of the leisure experience that are frequently associated with the experience of rest, as a possibility of continuing and deepening the experience of constructive leisure, namely absorption and psychological involvement.

ABSORPTION AND PSYCHOLOGICAL INVOLVEMENT

Absorption and engagement or involvement with the experience are qualities of leisure that are considered fundamental by some authors (Csikszentmihalyi & Csikszentmihalyi, 1998; Mannell & Kleiber, 1997; Tinsley & Tinsley, 1986). However, these are not the attributes most commonly found in research studies on everyday leisure experiences and even less so in modern-day ordinary leisure situations. Absorption and psychological involvement are experiences that demand a much greater level of attention and concentration than most people usually use in their everyday activities.

The psychological involvement of leisure is broken down in cognitive elements such as focused attention, affective elements such as increased sensitivity, and other more specific elements such as losing the awareness of time and forgetting about oneself. Cognitively what happens is a narrowing of the attention focus and a high degree of concentration on what is being experienced, be it a task, a situation, a scene, a person, or an object that is being observed. According to experts, this phenomenon means to get completely involved with the experience and it also manifests itself through the feeling of control over a given situation or decrease of self-consciousness and loss of the awareness of time.

Before we approach the subject of absorption proper, we have to add that the basis of this phenomenon is the presence of a certain level of interest, understood as the support to what is necessary and possible in terms of human action—that is, as an overall positive affect whose function is to stimulate behavior. This means that without interest an individual cannot do or learn how to do things because he is not sufficiently involved. Besides interest, excitement is an important and necessary factor in the psychological support to personal efforts, particularly in the long term, since without enthusiasm such efforts could not be achieved, let alone the required commitment.

These assumptions apply more clearly when we think of the experiences called *serious leisure* by Stebbins (1992). *Serious leisure* is leisure that can generate a long term commitment, requiring greater personal involvement. Involvement, in turn, depends on the meaning assigned to the action and, after some time, on the maintenance of a certain degree of excitement.

Concentration on the experience is considered by Csikszentmihalyi (1997) one of the most frequent flow experiences—consciousness flow—or optimal experiences. In this type of experience, the attention directed to the task at hand and to the present time is such that there is no room left in the mind for information that is not very relevant. However, we stress that a high degree of concentration should not be taken for automatism, although in some circumstances both may look similar at first sight. Absorption leads the individual, during the activity, to forget almost everything that does not have a direct relationship or that is not useful for what he is doing at the moment. This is why during leisure experiences of this type, the person involved in it does not think about the past or the future, neither is he concerned with his own image, his ego or with the passing of time.

Concentration at this level allows us to identify such a psychological commitment and personal dedication to the experience that the individual does not think about who is around him or about himself. During the ordinary course of our psychological functioning, the mental state can show episodes of entropy that invade the harmonious operation of the psychological energy. However, in optimal experiences the demands of the structured activity impose an order and exclude potential interferences by the disorder of consciousness.

Csikszentmihalyi (1997, pp. 95–98) explains that extraordinary experiences, and we might include among them some experiences of leisure and entertainment, imply "not being worried about losing control." It is not about having the actual control over the situation, but rather a perception of the *possibility of control* that enables the individual to get totally involved in what he is doing, mitigating fears and concerns. This phenomenon usually occurs more clearly in risk activities, even if it is a calculated risk, such as in adventure sports.

Tinsley and Tinsley (1986) establish a connection between the degree of concentration and the intensity and quality of the leisure and entertainment experience. For these authors, a high degree of concentration is associated with a quantitative and qualitative improvement in the perception of body sensations (what the authors call sensitivity) and in the perception of affective stimuli and emotional intensities. The enhancement of perception is related to everything that occurs within the experience, which sometimes also includes the environment. This helps us understand why leisure experiences in natural environments tend to provide moments of involvement with nature. Furthermore, Tinsley and Tinsley (1986) explain that by increasing the concentration on oneself and on the experience from a low to a moderate level, there is an increase in the power and quality of the experience. On the other hand, by increasing the concentration from a moderate to a high level, the power and quality of the subjective experience of leisure is reduced. However, these statements lack any concrete empirical proof.

In addition to the concentration on the activity, some studies of leisure experiences show that individuals become unselfconscious, what Csikszentmihalyi (1997) describes as "out of Self focus." Here I would like to dedicate a few lines to explain the difference between the concept of "self "and the concept of "I" as it is made in humanist, existential, and transpersonal psychology.

"I" corresponds to the structuring aspect of personality, which is more superficial and manageable; it could be compared to the concept of the "ego" from the psychoanalytical point of view; on the other hand, the "self" corresponds to an integrating center of meaning and generator of authenticity. In Jung's (1964) "individuation" processes, in Maslow's self-actualization, in Rogers' (1982) self-actualization and in Wilber's (1998) expansion of consciousness, people walk towards their personal development, towards the recognition of their self. The conception of self understood as such becomes important to show to what extent an individual can get involved with an experience of leisure. However, we do not want to state here that all experiences of leisure totally involve people, since the level of involvement can vary from person to person, and among different situations.

Some experiences of leisure involve involuntarily forgetting about oneself, in the sense of not paying attention to one's own needs, desires, thoughts or feelings during the activity. Obviously this is a situation that is restricted to a certain period of time that could last from seconds to many hours, during which we do not control the phenomenon, precisely because we are totally absorbed by it. The activity in these cases becomes automatic, with no role to be played by the "I" or by the ego. Sometimes a feeling of deep union with the surrounding environment, like a landscape, a team, or a community can come with the loss of self-consciousness. This type of feeling also shows the presence of a psychological involvement or absorption and results in a greater level of trust in oneself and in the circumstances or people involved.

Generally speaking, pleasant experiences with clear objectives, stable rules, and challenges that are in accordance with one's skills minimize the possibilities of threats to one's personality. Trust, in turn, is conducive to an even greater dedication or involvement without, however, leading to loss of control. "Loss of self-consciousness does not involve a loss of personality and, certainly, is not a loss of consciousness, just a loss of the consciousness of personality. What is under the threshold of consciousness is the concept of personality, the information we use to represent ourselves" (Csikszentmihalyi, 1997, p. 105).

Another manifestation that is characteristic of some experiences of leisure, in which there is psychological involvement and a high degree of concentration is the loss of the awareness of time. The individual perception of *time* during leisure experiences may not correspond to the real chronological or social time. Therefore, a person may easily forget the hands of the watch and enjoy the activity or situation as if time was not going by. On the other hand, we may qualify the experience of leisure regarding its duration, being either long or very short, slow or fast, having as a basis only associated subjective perceptions or perceptions caused by other factors inherent in the experience: enjoyment, relaxation, anxiety, and so on, particularly resulting from a *devotion* in physical and/or psychological terms.

What is most commonly found in experiences of leisure is the feeling that time goes by fast; however, the opposite may occur in activities in which time is essential, like participating in a race or in a marathon. However, studies on leisure do not clarify whether losing awareness of time is an attribute in itself or a direct consequence of the high degree of concentration.

It is evident that concentrating in the way described by Csikszentmihalyi (1998), Maslow (1999) and Tinsley and Tinsley (1986) is not a very common behavior in the hectic life of urban societies or, in other words, people are not trained to focus all their attention and energy on one single activity, particularly in their free time. Technologies enable us to perform many different tasks simultaneously. Additionally, people increasingly try to do more in less time, as if this was the optimal pattern to be followed. The real need of following this pattern or the quality of the results thus achieved is not often questioned. The fact is that the more we accelerate, the more difficult it becomes to have an experience of concentration and the psychological involvement in what we are doing.

Considering this reality, the experience of constructive leisure becomes even more important, because it is a way of exercising the ability of having psychological involvement, either through focused attention or the sensitive dedication to freely chosen activities.

INTROSPECTIVE STATES

Introspection is an attribute that is not widely investigated in the field of leisure studies, but nevertheless is something that becomes an inevitable experience for those who reach certain levels of maturity and psychological individuation. Personal development in this sphere generally leads to a capacity of deep personal search—intrapsychologically and spiritually—in which introspection is a necessary and often spontaneous exercise.

Introspection, closeness with oneself, and deep reflection are possible experiences in constructive leisure, particularly when the experience is associated with the appreciation of natural or artistic beauty. It should be highlighted here that the experience of closeness or introspection can acquire many different forms such as to stop and think about oneself, pray, meditate, contemplate, appreciate, etc. or be devoid of any specific form, and what is really fundamental is the psychological, cognitive and emotional state and/or the spiritual state of those having the experience.

The close contact with oneself is a challenge in the hypermodern society. "Few of us would seek to live in solitude, but who would not like to be alone for a while?" (Servan-Schreiber, 2001, p. 24). Moreno (1994) states that this practice is not sufficiently valued and it is possibly the result of an education focused on results and outputs.

In humanist psychology, *solitude* is understood as a vital need, as important as being and sharing with other people. For Jourard and Landsman (1987), the reason of solitude is evident, since when we see ourselves separate from others and remain silent, we have the opportunity to reflect and appreciate what could be our own perspective in relation to so many stimuli and opinions that reach us. This solitude does not equate with depriving oneself from the company of other people, because it is a freely chosen solitude. Leisure, in some cases, may mean the opportunity to be alone and enjoy solitude, particularly if we consider life in urban centers where we must have opportunities to be alone and thus connect to our own selves.

There are specific and recognized experiences that facilitate this close contact with oneself and that can happen through more or less structured methods, which are always related to a considerable level of relaxation as, for example, yoga, meditation, prayer, contemplation of nature, and the like. The experience of relaxation can clear our ideas and correct values, in that it frees us from automatic behaviors.

Relaxation in deeper levels and performed frequently is a gate for self-discovery, since the individual is freed from his mental habits and automatisms, diving into a state of inner silence and calm. Fontcuberta (1976) adds: "when there is silence, rest, emptiness, something resonates inside like the awareness of oneself" (p. 47).

Naranjo (1991), when writing on the psychology of meditation, says that meditating, in almost all techniques, means to stimulate the focused attention on an imaginary or real object, with the symbolic function of recalling the center of the individual or the core of their being, the *self*. From this point of view, we can understand the technical proposition of meditation of "*concentrating*" or focusing on oneself since one of the objectives of meditation is to get to know oneself.

In some eastern philosophies, *oneself* corresponds to an abstraction of the emptiness or *sunyata* (bottomless). Based on this idea, eastern thinkers believe that the experience of *nirvana* (Buddhist) or of the *fana-fillah* (Islamic) is nothing but the "awakening to reality and finding one's own identity in the emptiness that holds all things" (Naranjo, 1991, p. 34). In this reality, eastern philosophies describe the experience of transcendence through deep self-reflection, with which it is possible to contact the deepest parts of the *being* (Daly, Lancee, & Polivy, cited in Argyle, 1992).

These experiences are usually facilitated by music, reading, or an environment of natural beauty, depending on the type of person and circumstance. Theoretically we find that the experience of introspection and the encounter with oneself is not such a rare phenomenon if we consider the human potential to achieve it. However, we do not know if in our everyday life, with the urban lifestyle that prevails among us, we can have the internal and external conditions for this type of experience to happen.

Eastern philosophies are not the only sources of thinking that value and propose experiences of introspection, self-reflection and transcendence. If we understand *transcendence* in its multiple meanings, as supported by Maslow (1999), then transcendence will not really look as something rare to us. According to Maslow (1999), we can find transcendence when we lose the sensation of being observed, tending to introspection and observation of our own behavior, when we feel affection for those who no longer live, and when we work for future generations (temporal transcendence). Additionally, it also refers to the transcendence of culture, of one's own past, of selfishness or egocentrism, transcendence of pain, transcendence of the polarity between "we–they" and of dichotomies, transcendence of the basic needs—that is, through satisfaction or renunciation—transcendence of the opinion of others, of one's own weaknesses and dependencies, transcendence of the present and concrete reality, and even the experience of the "mystic merge with another person, with the whole cosmos" or with nature (Maslow, 1999, pp. 321–333). However, above all, Maslow (1999) states that transcendence is nothing but a human ability to excel, meaning "doing more than we believed we could do or more than we have done in the past" (Maslow, 1999, p. 327).

Christian tradition, in turn, suggests that the experiences of *prayer* and *contemplation* serve as a contrast to everyday life; that is, they offer the possibility of experiencing transcendence, as suggested by Saint Benedict (in Gabiña Aizpuru, 1999): "*ora et labora.*" Gabiña Aizpuru (1999) interprets Saint Benedict by saying that work represents the earthly and profane dimension of human activity, while prayer and contemplation represent a manifestation of the sacred dimension or a time dedicated to the divine in us. However, neither Saint Benedict nor Aizpuru try to overvalue a dimension at the expense of the other, but rather present them as complementary and equally important for the integrity of humans.

Additionally, the essence of the experience of Christian introspection as proposed both by Saint Benedict and Saint Ignatius and other personalities from history is the attitude of listening and the experience of receptivity, although people sometimes interpret prayer as a monolog. For Gabiña Aizpuru,

> prayer... will be pleasurable if he who is praying is not so concerned with his rituals, ideas or feelings, which could lead him to the distraction of egocentrism, but rather submerge into the serene and pleasant leisure of putting himself before God and listen to His Word, being sure that it will come. (Gabiña Aizpuru, 1999, p. 219)

Therefore, we understand that free time and leisure can be the time and space for the divine in people and that introspection or the encounter with oneself, with nature, or with beauty in the form of contemplation is an expression of the most sublime aspects of the human being. Therefore, experiences of profound introspection, of psychological or spiritual nature can be experiences of leisure, as well put by Godbey (1989): "The nature of leisure is subjective and dialectic. The behavior of leisure is ultimately unlimited, non-rational and full of meaning which is, or can be, totally spiritual" (p. 157). Benson and Dossey (in Saint-Arnaud, 2002) also talk about experiences of prayer and contemplation as experiences associated with some level of relaxation and that converge in psychophysical concentration, in the attitude of attention regarding an inner presence, in the ability we have to get away from the distractions that prevent us from calming our body, emotions, and mind.

By studying the experiences of introspection in its distinct forms, we find that the elements that constitute the experiences of leisure are often interrelated and complementary. For example, the experience of relaxation and encounter with oneself cannot be reached if the individual does not get psychologically involved and let himself get absorbed by the experience. This is not very different from what happens in experiences of encounters with nature and beauty, as we will see next.

ENCOUNTERS WITH NATURE AND BEAUTY

The attitude of looking inside oneself does not take place only in experiences such as meditation, prayer, or other practices based on the "art of relaxed concentration" (Gabiña Aizpuru, 1999, p. 42) can also evoke feelings of well-being, peace, calm, and quiet, as is the case with contemplation of art and nature. Along the line of personal experiences with leisure of more receptive, introspective, and reflexive nature, we will talk a little about the relationships of humans with *nature* and with *beauty*, which translate in a very particular way what constructive leisure can be.

We all know that contact with nature favors contemplative and reflexive states. According to Jourard and Landsman (1987), contact with the natural physical world—beaches, mountains, parks, fields, animals and plants—has the ability to provide us with a sense of peace that is very different than that experienced by people who live in urban and industrialized settings. This type of experience reminds us of the fact that we do not have just a body, but rather a body that is made up of the same elements we find in nature and which also belong to us. These authors add that chronic physical strains and the accelerated paces in talking and moving are more commonly found in people who live separated from their own nature and from the nature that surrounds them.

Cuenca (2000) states the existence of an environmental–ecological dimension in leisure, recognizing in it the value and importance of the environment and nature for the personal experience of leisure in a humanist conception. The appreciation of nature and its relationship with the divine and with things of the spirit was clearer in ancient societies, when poems and chants expressed the importance of nature to people, to their personal formation and happiness.

> It is difficult to explain any experience of leisure separated from its environment.... Sometimes, however, the context is no longer a complementary element of the experience and constitutes its core, its main reason.... One could say that the environmental–ecological dimension of leisure is the disinterested satisfaction resulting from the encounter with the desired environment, while the activity that generates such satisfaction is not necessarily important. (Cuenca, 2003, p. 125)

Cuenca (2003) also points to the possibility of developing the awareness of environmental conservation and preservation through encounters with nature, which can take place through rural or ecological tourism. Today it is not uncommon to find people who talk about the value of nature and who support environmental positions, but this will not necessarily mean that people will recognize the interdependence and the complementary character of the relationship between humans and nature; more studies are needed that go deeper into this subject and describe the specific contents of this relationship, going beyond the appreciation of beautiful landscapes.

Some studies on leisure suggest that the personal enjoyment experience is often easier when people get close to nature, live with it, and learn from it, whether they are conscious of this relationship or not. A study conducted at the White River National Forest in Colorado by Hull, Stewart, and Young Yi (1992) showed that subjects were more susceptible to the fact of walking in one or another direction as a function of their location in the park. Those who were going up were more satisfied than those who were going down; that is, the significant interactions among the location of the signs intentionally used during the experiment, in addition to the direction of the trip, also affected the excitement, relaxation, and scenic beauty identified by the trekkers.

Another finding was that a high degree of scenic beauty increased the feelings of satisfaction, although trekkers who were returning seemed less sensitive to external factors and focused more on internal factors such as fatigue. They also found that trekkers were not looking for a static outcome in recreation, such as solitude or satisfaction, but rather a wider range of feelings such as relaxation with peaks of excitement. Ultimately, the conclusion was that the patterns of experience in nature documented by the trekkers suggest that people can feel excited or slightly activated and relaxed all at the same time.

According to Saint-Arnaud (2002), the beauty of nature is a source of pleasure to people. While we contemplate a sunset or a lake, harmony—a quality of nature—invades us, causing a calming resonance. Its reverberations can transform an attitude, even if one is not aware of this possibility. For Tinsley (1988), the appreciation of the aesthetic qualities of the activity or of its environment which manifests itself through contemplation seems to be associated with the relationship between people and the environment, which the author calls *aesthetic experience*. Tinsley (1988) states that people need aesthetic experiences and intellectual stimulation, which he considers a benefit that leisure can provide.

The subjective condition of an aesthetic experience is the contemplative state in relation to an object, the action of entering into its world in a specific state of consciousness. Maslow (1999) distinguishes the aesthetic perception or attitude from other psychological processes, because the former savors, appreciates, and enjoys without interfering or controlling. The end result of aesthetic perception "is the complete inventory of the precept, in which everything can be equally savored and in which we tend to abandon the assessments conditioned by greater or lesser importance. Here we look for a greater wealth in precept" (Maslow, 1999, p. 97).

We would like to highlight here the intimist, subjective, and emotionally positive nature of aesthetic experiences, be it due to a gift of nature or some human expression such as the arts. Amigo (2000) proposes that the aesthetic view takes place when we break with ordinary interpretation and there are unanswered questions, i.e., when we allow things to surprise and move us. The aesthetic attitude, like most psychological experiences, may vary and coexist with other phenomena, but it is characterized by understanding and enjoyment.

Art, in particular, is a human phenomenon that privileges the relationship of an aesthetic nature, because works of art, either from plastic arts, music, theater or literature, invites us to sensitively look at and listen to things. In this sense, appreciation or contemplation of art or, better said, of the beauty one sees in it, sometimes is a deep leisure experience.

Kant (1973) said that the work of art is a gratifying occupation "in itself and in its own sake," where the aesthetic pleasure is a disinterested pleasure that flows in the realm of sensitivity. According to Amigo (2000), this concept of aesthetic experience reflects the autotelic humanist leisure.

According to the author, frequently "the aesthetic judgment is followed by an intention of universal validation" (p. 61). Nevertheless, if the agreement of others regarding my own aesthetic judgment does takes place, this is because they too were satisfied, not because some sort of intellectual consensus has been reached, since the aesthetic judgment is, above all, disinterested and not previously determined by concepts and rules. According to Amigo, "this aspiration for universal validation separates the beautiful and the pleasant, because regarding the latter, every individual has his own taste. Therefore, the universal capacity of communicating a state of mind in a given representation is based on taste judgment" (Amigo, 2000, p. 99).

Beauty can mediate the relationship between sensitivity and reason, and for this reason it manifests itself as a necessary human condition. For Amigo (2000), in understanding the beautiful, what matters does not possess it, but rather the *encounter* that takes place "when there is a fit between an involving reality and the subject that immerses into it" (p. 103). The primitive task of the aesthetic experience is stressed as "the capacity to take a leap from the objective level to the playful level." This change of perspective in looking at reality, according to the theory of leisure, can be understood as one of its characteristic elements, as changing a chip or taking a quantum leap, using a post-modern language. It is another form of transcendence, the experience of transcending to conditionings that are inherent in the ordinary and accelerated life in hypermodern times. In this process, the material elements and physical events acquire another, non-utilitarian meaning: *the splendor of beauty.*

In the aesthetic encounter, on the one hand, the individual feels the joy and enthusiasm generated when contemplating the shape, wealth of shades, and expressive intensity of a reality. On the other hand, it plays with his creative capacity which is, for the artist, the source of meaning and enjoyment. We think that such experience of *encounter,* as presented by Amigo, also takes place in the close relationship between people and nature, since the latter also makes us sensitively look at and listen to things, inviting us to contemplate them without possessing them.

A profound encounter with oneself, with nature, and with beauty implies sensations and feelings related to what is most human in people: openness, enjoyment, harmony, peace, and serenity, which manifest themselves particularly in true experiences of constructive leisure. We have had a chance to take a look at theories on some subjective phenomena related to experiences of constructive leisure. These are examples that show that constructive leisure in people's lives can be used to prevent stress and promote a better quality of life.

Overall, leisure, as well as some forms of entertainment, consists of psychosocial attributes that, when combined, make every experience unique. Although the attributes of leisure most commonly identified by individuals are the perception of freedom, the intrinsic meaning or motivation, enjoyment, the interpersonal encounter, and rest, we think it is important to know other attributes that have been highlighted here, such as distraction and rupture, absorption and psychological involvement, introspection, transcendence, and aesthetic appreciation.

In this regard, we saw that the psychosocial phenomena involved in experiences of leisure, looked at from a humanist point of view, cross the barriers of social elements, turning an individual into the protagonist of his experiences of leisure and through them of this own quality of life. This knowledge becomes important as we can relate it to broader and more practical aspects of life, such as personal and family well-being, the quality of professional performance, quality of life, and satisfaction with one's life. Therefore, I would like to close this chapter by looking at the social dimension of leisure.

According to Cuenca (2000), the way of life of modern society has negative effects on people, particularly with the increase in the level of stress, development of unhealthy habits, and the loss of stable models. In this context, leisure acquires a preventive role necessary for the restructuring of the physical and mental balance, and consequently, it has a direct impact on the quality of life.

A proper practice of leisure could cut the costs spent to treat chemical addiction, depression, juvenile violence, and family conflicts. Many of these problems are related to the lack of experiences of constructive leisure, that is, to free time that is characterized by lack of meaning, by existential emptiness, and by the boredom of being a mere spectator. To these examples we would add consumerist leisure, escapist activism, and the compulsive search for fleeting sensations and instant pleasures.

Csikszentmihalyi (1997) relates enjoyment with quality of life and happiness, pointing to two ways to enhance them: the first would be to try to act upon the external conditions so that they match our goals and, secondly, we should change our experiences vis-à-vis the external conditions in order to adapt them to our goals. Anyway, Csikszentmihalyi (1997) recognizes that the strategies to improve quality of life and make us get closer to happiness do not work in isolation. Therefore, we can understand quality of life and happiness, regarding leisure, as depending both on external conditions and on every individual's experiences. In other words, working for a better offer of activities and for access to leisure can help, but this alone will not guarantee the experience of constructive leisure and let alone a better quality of life. The way in which every individual perceives and thinks time itself, free time, and experiences of leisure is as important as the content of these experiences. Leisure is related to happiness and quality of life in that it is based on a humanist ethics; that is, it is an experience that brings benefits to oneself and to others, so that we can find ways of achieving satisfaction without harming anyone.

We believe that there are different ways to live in the same social economic and cultural context. Although conditions might be similar, the attitude adopted when facing these conditions, the perception of space and time, what every individual values and prioritizes, the personal view or the subjective experience of leisure can make quality of life and satisfaction in life very different among people who are seemly close. It is a matter of becoming aware of the transforming potential of one's own choices.

Humanist and existentialist influences are clear on the concepts and theoretical and empirical assumptions presented here, and this could not be any different, since talking about leisure as a personal experience is only possible from the appreciation of the human elements that reflect on all spheres of the analysis: the human character that exists in the social reality, in culture, in politics, and the economy. From a scientific point of view, there is a tendency to fragment objects and remove them from the context that gives them a shape or from the content that gives them meaning, respectively, from humanity or the human character, something we modestly tried to overcome here by recognizing the subjective elements of the experiences of free time and leisure and their relationship with life as whole.

REFERENCES

Amigo, M.L. (2000). *El arte como vivencia de ocio.* Bilbao, Spain: Universidad de Deusto.

Argyle, M.L. (1992). *La psicología de la felicidad.* Madrid, Spain: Alianza.

Boff, L. (2002). *Experimentar Deus: A transparência de todas as coisas.* Campinas, Brasil: Verus.

Csikszentmihalyi, M. (1997). *Fluir: Una psicología de la felicidad.* Barcelona, Spain: Kairós.

Csikszentmihalyi, M., & Csikszentmihalyi, S. (1998). *Experiencia Óptima: Estudios psicológicos del flujo en la conciencia.* Bilbao, Spain: Desclee de Brower.

Cuenca, C.M. (Ed.). (2000). *Ocio y desarrollo humano. Propuestas para el 6° Congreso Mundial de Ocio.* Bilbao, Spain: Universidad de Deusto.

Cuenca, C.M. (2003). *Ocio humanista: Dimensiones y manifestaciones actuales del ocio.* Documentos de Estudios de Ocio núm.6. Bilbao, Spain: Universidad de Deusto.

Dumazedier, J. (1964). *Hacia una civilización del ocio.* Barcelona, Spain: Estela.

Fontcuberta, A.B. (1976). *Relajación y energía.* Barcelona, Spain: Elicien.

Gabiña Aizpuru, S. (1999). *La sociedad del ocio y la religión.* Madrid, Spain: San Pablo.

Godbey, G. (1989). *Leisure in your life: An exploration* (5th ed.). State College, PA: Venture Publishing.

Godbey, G., & Robinson, J. (1997). *Time for life. The surprising ways Americans use their time.* University Park, PA: Pennsylvania State University Press.

Hull, R. B., Stewart, W. P., & Young Yi, K. (1992). Experience patterns: Capturing the dynamic nature of a recreation experience. *Journal of Leisure Research, 24*(3), 240–252.

Jourard, S.M., & Landsman, T. (1987). *La personalidad saludable: El punto de vista de la psicologia humanística.* Mexico: Trillas.

Jung, C. G. (1964). *O homem e os seus símbolos.* Rio de Janeiro, Brasil: Nova Fronteira.

Kant, M. (1973). *Critica del juicio, Libro I, Sección I.* Madrid, Spain: Espassa Colpe.

Lipovetsky, G. (2004). *Tempos hipermodernos.* São Paulo, Brasil: Barcarolla.

Mannell, R.C., & Kleiber, D.A. (1997). *A social psychology of leisure.* State College, PA: Venture Publishing.

Maslow, A. (1999). *La personalidad creadora.* Barcelona, Spain: Kairós.

Moreno, I. (1994). *Todos tenemos tiempo.Nueva práctica del tiempo libre en el siglo XXI.* Buenos Aires, Argentina: Humanitas.

Naranjo, C. (1991). *Psicologia da meditação.* São Paulo: Instituto Thame.

Pascal, B. (1979). *Pensamentos.* São Paulo, Brasil: Abril Cultural.

Rhoden, I. (2004). *Experiencias Personales de Ocio: desarrollo de una herramienta para la identificación de sus cualidades subjetivas.* Doctoral dissertation, Instituto de Estudios de Ocio, Universidad de Deusto, Bilbao, Spain.

Rogers, C.R. (1982). *El proceso de convertirse en persona.* (L. R. Wainberg, Trans.). Barcelona, Spain: Ediciones Paidos.

Saint-Arnaud, Y. (2002). *La guérison par le plaisir.* Ottawa, Canada: Novalis, Université Saint-Paul.

Schultz, J.H. (1969). *El entrenamiento Autógeno.* Barcelona, Spain: Editorial Científico-Médica.

Servan-Schreiber, J.L. (2001). *El nuevo arte de vivir el tiempo. Contra el estrés.* Barcelona, Spain: Paidós.

Stebbins, R.A. (1992). *Amateurs, professionals and serious leisure.* Montreal, Quebec, Canada: McGill-Queens University Press.

Tinsley, H. E. A. (1988). The psychological benefits of leisure counseling, *Society and Leisure, 7*(1), 125–140.

Tinsley, H. E. A., & Tinsley, D. J. (1986). A theory of the attributes, benefits, and causes of leisure experience, *Leisure Sciences, 8*(1), 1–45.

Tinsley, H. E. A., Tinsley, D. J., Hinson, J. & Holt, M. (1993). Attributes of leisure and works experiences, *Journal of Counseling Psychology, 40*(4), 447–455.

Wilber, K.A. (1998). Consciência sem fronteiras—Pontos de vista do oriente e do ocidente sobre o crescimento pessoal (10th ed.). São Paulo, Brasil: Cultrix.

SECTION IV

EXAMINING THE BIGGER PICTURE OF OCCUPATIONAL HEALTH AND WELL BEING

CHAPTER 11

"NOT SO FAST, MY FRIEND!"

The Eternal Marital Bliss or Imminent Divorce of Leadership and Neuroscience

Thomas A. Zeni, M. Ronald Buckley, and Anthony C. Klotz
University of Oklahoma

Milorad M. Novicevic
University of Mississippi

ABSTRACT

Due to the potential breakthroughs associated with understanding psychological phenomena via measurement of physiological processes, there has been growing impetus among organizational researchers to adopt these methodologies and measures in the organization science discipline, including leadership. However, upon more thorough investigation, physiological measurement and analysis is fraught with a number of unsettling and unresolved issues that threaten the validity of the potential psychological inferences drawn from this type of research. Here, we identify these threats to validity as they pertain to the study of leadership by first highlighting the shortcomings of physiology-to-psychology research. Next, based on current

Coping and Prevention, pages 195–217

> knowledge, we argue that these physiological tools, while valuable for many areas, are not appropriate for addressing those areas in leadership that have been identified as the most critical research areas of future investigations in leadership at this time.

Biological science has long been a sister science to the study of psychological phenomena. Often, the study of biological processes can be used to inform or increase our understanding of human behavior and of how the brain functions (i.e., how people think), and, in turn, expand our understanding of psychology as a whole. Developments in technology (specifically MRI, fMRI, and PET scans) have drawn heightened interest to examining brain processes from a biological standpoint and attempting to tie these processes to psychological phenomena such as cognition, emotion, attitudes, behavior, and learning, among other areas.

Of course, the "family" created by joining biological and psychological sciences must continue to grow. In fact, it only seems natural that the biological sciences, through one of its most popular offspring, neuroscience, would pair with one of psychological science's most popular offspring, organizational science, specifically within the fertile area of leadership studies. This is reminiscent of the colonial practice in the American colonies and Western European countries called bundling. Bundling was the traditional practice of wrapping one person in a bed accompanied by another, usually as a part of courting behavior with nary a board between them. Instead of bundling two people, however, we seem to be in the early, awkward stages of bundling leadership and neuroscience and hoping the impending nuptials will be successful, supplying information and fecundity.

Cross-discipline relationships in which one side of the dyad is the organizational sciences, however, are often rockier than those between myriad other areas. Often with organizational sciences, researchers must balance the passionate desire of intellectual pursuit with the frigidity of pragmatic application. In other words, the marriage of neuroscience and leadership studies must, like good relationships, strike many compromises between the needs of both parties. It is in this thought that the future of this union becomes dubitable.

Speaking plainly, the extent to which biological science and leadership studies provides a productive area of exploration depends greatly upon the utility of this exploration to organizations. Whereas this line of research is undeniably intriguing, a closer examination of the current state of affairs, particularly with respect to neuroscience, raises several questions that must be considered when attempting to evaluate the usefulness of biological studies within the organizational leadership domain. As scientists and practitioners, we feel it is important to raise awareness to these concerns and will highlight them from multiple perspectives.

We certainly do not suggest that neuroscientific research is lacking in merit, intrigue, or potential value to leadership research. Our basic concern (and largely tied to its popularity and intrigue) is that applications rooted in this approach may be potentially misleading, and through popularization, overzealously adopted within organizational practice (Weisberg, 2008). Indeed, empirical research demonstrates that simply adding neuroscience-based criteria to either good or bad explanations of psychological phenomena positively increases layperson judgments of the veracity of such findings (Weisberg, Keil, Godstein, Rawson, & Gray, 2008).

The addition of biological evidence to our existing research should be considered a welcome and interesting area of exploration, yet significant danger exists in the sense that burgeoning fields may be subject to overpopularization prior to the necessary rigorous testing. In a venue with real-world consequences (i.e., organizational sciences and leadership studies), it is our responsibility to stem the effects of mainstream popularity, lest we allow the valuable input of biological research to become a flavor-of-the-day, pop-like phenomenon. In this instance specifically, organizational leaders, the consumers of our knowledge, already have their hands full distinguishing between executive coaches versus intramural coaches, results from personality tests versus results from Facebook questionnaires, and team-building exercises versus exercises that merely waste valuable team resources.

Thus, the purpose of this chapter is twofold. First, we take a critical look at the methodological shortcomings of physiological research to assuage the unbridled enthusiasm surrounding its extension to organizational science. Second, we examine the most pressing leadership research issues through the lens of these physiological methods to propose whether these tools can add value to leadership research where scholars believe it is most needed. That is, physiological measures may well be able to answer questions related to leadership in organizations, but are these questions ones that need to be asked, or is it simply a case of the methodological tail wagging the knowledge-seeking dog?

So, in considering the scientist/practitioner perspectives, we highlight several concerns with the current state of neurological research from a methodological stance. While elaborating on the relationship between two scientific domains (both of which have matured independently), it appears both logical and prudent to take lessons from established relationships in order to minimize growing pains. Therefore, our discussion of neuroscience and leadership includes reflections on existing relationships between neuroscience and other domains, as well as considerations from prior links between organizational science and biological sciences.

THE MARRIAGE LICENSE: ARE THESE MEASURES VALID?

Just as the marriage license is a necessary but insufficient condition for a successful marriage, validity is the minimum price of entry for new measures and methods in the organizational sciences. Our primary concern with the integration of neuroscience and leadership is the apparent lack of consistent methodological rigor and the absence of standardized, accepted practices within neuroscience. The appeal of neuroscience relies largely on the premise that this field will enable "hard science" and measurement (via neurological research) to inform theory and practice of "soft skills," such as leadership (Ringleb & Rock, 2008). However, threats to the validity of conclusions drawn from neurological research abound. Specifically, the methods and statistical analyses employed within the domain raise serious doubts as to the efficacy of including neuroscientific findings within the organizational science domain.

Neuroscientific studies operate under a general set of guiding principles. Foremost is the idea that brain activity is localized; specific areas or regions of the brain carry out specific activities, functions, and so forth. Through this central tenet comes the idea that specific human behaviors and psychological processes are also localized, or controlled by specific areas of the brain. Brain imaging techniques effectively measure activation of localized areas of the brain before, and subsequently during, the activation of a specific behavior and/or psychological process. The brain is divided into cellular level units of measurement known as voxels. Individual voxels are examined for activation, typically derived from increased blood and/or oxygen flow, and areas of activated voxels are identified, typically in localized clusters. These clusters are then labeled as regions of interest (ROI), which become the focal point for study when eliciting a specific behavior or psychological process.

This basic model of neuroscientific practice has become institutionalized within the research stream and has been improved upon over the years by rapid advances in technology. As one might imagine, measuring the activation of individual cells across time, and then aggregating these data in some form, produces an incredibly huge number of individual data points for analysis. It is here, in the statistical analysis of these data points, that the need for caution emerges, both within the neuroscience literature (Kriegeskorte, Lindquist, Nichols, Poldrack, & Vul, 2010; Kriegeskorte, Simmons, Bellgowan, & Bake, 2009; Vul, Harris, Winkielman, & Pashler, 2009) and in other research domains seeking to be informed by neuroscientific practice.

The need for caution in these analyses is an empirical issue, but one that potentially invalidates the conclusions drawn from this type of data. Because ROI (and individual voxels) are identified by applying some manipulation, and then further examined as the effect of that manipulation, the analyses are circular or non-independent. Explaining an observation in terms of itself adds to this notion of circularity. Furthermore, many inferential statistical analyses operate under an assumption of independent data; that is, observations from one data set are independent of the data set to which it is compared. Clearly, identifying an ROI and then comparing activation of voxels within that ROI across manipulated conditions seems to be a violation of this assumption. This practice effectively represents the gathering of mass amounts of data, and then "cherry-picking" the data based on desired outcomes. As researchers, we must therefore be wary of any conclusions drawn from this biased type of analysis.

This type of selective analysis has the consummate effect of introducing a form of selection bias (Kriegeskorte et al., 2009) into the data, distorting point estimates and confusing conclusions of inferential analysis. The perils of selection bias are well known within the organizational sciences domain, and in spite of the allure of neuroscientific data, we must continue to maintain current standards of methodological rigor. Unfortunately, neuroscience, albeit in an earlier stage of paradigm development, has not always adhered to these standards.

In a review of published studies across top-level journals within the neuroscientific domain, Kriegeskorte et al. (2009) report that out of 134 studies since 2008, 42% contained analyses that violated the independence assumption, and potentially another 14% may have violated this assumption but insufficient methodological detail in the reporting prevented a definitive determination. While the effect of this violation is indeterminable without examining or replicating the original data sets (Kriegeskorte et al., 2009), it has the potential to be quite large (covering well over 50% of the studies) and might drastically alter the findings of any given study. It is, at the least, a call for pause when drawing conclusions based on a neuroscientific study. Additionally, due to the apparent pervasive nature of these violations, it provides a significant reason for potentially limiting the association of organizational science's domain with neurological sciences, at least in its current state of methodological rigor.

Kriegeskorte et al. (2009) demonstrated the outcomes associated with violating independence assumptions using common neuroscience practices. They conclude that the effects of circularity are widespread, and influence data weighting, sorting, and selection, thus distorting results and invalidating statistical tests, even in the face of various statistical controls (such as correcting for multiple comparisons, controlling family-wise error rates, etc.). The idea is that corrupt data remain deficient even when treated with acceptable statistical controls. After demonstrating these effects, they call for a universal policy to be adopted within the neuroscientific domain regarding the treatment and elimination of circular data analyses. As outsiders to the neuroscience domain, we see this as a sound and logical clarion call—one that is drastically needed before other disciplines (such as the organizational sciences) should be comfortable fully embracing a collaborative, cross-disciplinary relationship and accepting, without question, conclusions drawn from neurological studies.

This particular debate continues among experts in the neurological science domain. In a review article, Kriegeskorte et al. (2010) revisit the discussion of circularity and its effect upon the neuroscience field. Several prominent authors address direct questions regarding the impact of circular analyses both on brain-mapping (identifying voxels) and estimating effects (based on ROI). The consensus across those interviewed reveals that (1) circularity is indeed a pervasive problem within the field, (2) circular analyses prevent obtaining usable estimates of effect sizes, (3) independent data sets are necessary before inferences from samples to the population can be made, and (4) inferences based on circular analyses are not statistically sound and should not be published without proper disclaimers and admonition that results are, until properly replicated, exploratory in nature (Kriegeskorte et al., 2010).

In these terms, organizational researchers can once again easily tie the dangers of this type of analysis to something we are already familiar with, and are critical of in our domain. We've already discussed the selection bias parallel, and in addition, Kriegeskorte and peers (2010) address the need for separation between exploratory and confirmatory data analysis—a well-known and discussed topic in the organizational sciences. Within our field, for example, a study that uses the same data set for both an exploratory and confirmatory factor analysis (for example) would come under scrutiny. If the data set were partitioned and examined independently, this would be acceptable; however, if the dataset were examined twice, once to build a model and once to test it (cross-validating a sample with the same sample), we would find this askew with accepted methodological standards and deem the study to be fatally flawed.

The same prudence/caution must be taken when considering results for neuroscientific studies in order to maintain the integrity of research findings within our field. Researchers interviewed by Kriegeskorte and colleagues (2010) appear to diverge slightly on both their opinions toward and tolerance of circularity depending on its use in brain mapping versus effect-size estimation. Circularity appears to be of less concern to brain-mapping efforts, where statistical controls (such as correcting for error rates, etc.) typically do a sufficient job of stemming the effects of the violation. That is, it is uncommon for a brain area to be identified as an active region when it is not. Whereas this may appear to be some good news, it is also clear that the experts' consensus suggests there is greater value in identifying effect sizes, such as how strongly a particular brain region activates in response to a phenomenon, than in mapping per se (Kriegeskorte et al., 2010). Indeed, it stands to reason that without measure of effect sizes, neuroscientific exploration is reduced to brain-mapping and akin to modern-day phrenology, the utility of which, particularly to organizational sciences, would appear trivial, at best.

On a similar note, even within brain-mapping practices, identification of activated voxels, and subsequently ROIs, depends on the somewhat arbitrary assignment of threshold values when determining activation states (Alferink & Farmer-Dougan, 2010). It is through the setting of a threshold value that localization is determined. Therefore, the results of studies and the determination of a localized region depend on the threshold value. Lower-level brain processes (such as sensory and motor processes) are known to be highly localized, with localization becoming more distributive as processes become more complex (Cacioppo, Lorig, Berntson, Norris, Rickett, & Nusbaum, 2003).

For complex social interactions, such as leadership, the threshold value used to identify significant versus insignificant voxels has become increasingly arbitrary. For example, behavioral differences may result from small variations in activated regions, and these variations may be well below the significance threshold and thus never identified. The system is far too complex and not understood well enough for us to be comfortable with assumptions of threshold values in many cases. Indeed, most cortical areas have been shown to serve multiple functions, and potentially to adapt when necessary, further calling into question the assumptions of localization that guide the use of measurement thresholds in neuroscientific research, particularly with respect to complex processes (Cacioppo et al., 2003).

Setting a threshold too high may lead to false assumptions of localization, and fail to capture areas of the brain that may be important in a particular phenomenon, and differences in thresholds across experiments or conditions must be considered when examining and interpreting results from such studies (Alferink & Farmer-Dougan, 2010). We would suggest that one unique contribution of this chapter is the revelation of a virtually unrecognized Achilles' heel of social neuroscience which lies in the arbitrary assignment of a threshold level that forces some degree of reliance on the localization assumption. This claim is grounded in the assumption that no single area of the brain is responsible for complex actions/thought.

Finally, it is important when considering neurological methods not to lose sight of the fact that current techniques in neuroscience simply correlate brain activity with behaviors, and do not necessarily imply any direct causality (Alferink & Farmer-Dougan, 2010). It is a mantra well rehearsed by the organizational science community (correlation does not equal causality). In the absence of more sophisticated technology and research methods, we can do no more than to understand that brain activity in a particular region is associated with a behavior, a psychological process, or a psychological phenomenon.

For example, it is undetermined as to whether or not behavior causes activation, activation causes behavior, or some other factor is responsible for both. This leads to a quandary concerning which is the predictor variable and which is the criterion variable. This shortcoming severely limits conclusions or the recommendations made based on neurological information. Lessons from the pairing of molecular biology to neuroscience highlight these issues. Genetic markers, much like activated brain areas, are only part of the puzzle involved when explaining complex behaviors (Lederhendler & Schulkin, 2000). This "systems perspective" of molecular biology reminds us that enabling of a behavior is not the same as determining or causing it, and that both nature and nurture might play an important role in this relationship.

Researchers need to understand more fully the workings of human biology before reliably drawing conclusions. In a recent discussion of several current trends in psychological exploration, Kagan (2007) highlights some of the concerns that rise from proceeding too quickly. Specifically, the author notes that psychologists incorporate multiple sources of measurement without fully understanding them or whether or not the sources are compatible. This issue is illustrated through developments/trends in neuroscience and genetics research. Technological advances in neuroscience have allowed psychologists to attempt to tie common psychological constructs, such as fear, to neuroscientific measurement. However, the trend has been to seek specific, localized brain areas in which activation is measured and called "fear." Similarly, advances in genetic research have prompted psychologists to seek specific alleles (one of a series of different forms of a gene) as predictive causes of specific behaviors or behavioral patterns.

In both cases, localization of brain function and genetic phenotype, complex biological functioning is often oversimplified in an attempt to explain a complex psychological phenomenon. For example, experiencing fear may elicit activation in the amygdala, but this does not mean the amygdala is the only area of the brain that handles fear, or that the handling of fear is the only function of the amygdala. Also, no specific allele or entire genome for that matter independently predicts an individual's mood or personality (Kagan, 2007). Furthermore, we now know that new ventures are more likely among those with higher testosterone levels (White, Thornhill, & Hampson, 2007). But is the testosterone level a causal factor of the new venture creation, a result of the new venture creation, or related to a third variable that is related to both testosterone production and new venture creation? Take your pick, but we cannot have it all three ways!

AFTER THE HONEYMOON: PRAGMATIC CONCERNS

Once newlyweds return from their honeymoon, the reality of living together sinks in, and the challenges associated with daily life together become real. Organizational research carries with it the burden of producing both solid scientific theories as well as guiding practice and application in a dynamic, real-world environment. For leadership studies, the real-world environment consists of particularly high stakes, and therefore the utility of the research domain, including both theory and application, must be carefully evaluated by the organizations it seeks to benefit. In a world where ROI means return on investment, and not region of interest, pragmatic concerns cannot be ignored. Early research pairing neuroscience and leadership appears to be quite intriguing, but it also raises a number of questions that should be answered before the two may successfully help us understand tomorrow's captains of industry.

The possibility of neuroscience fueling leadership, at least from an applied perspective, may lie in the concept of neuroplasticity. Neuroplasticity refers to the fact that the brain, with all its synapses, pathways, and complexities, can change. The human brain continuously changes and reorganizes itself to accommodate new information. While this phenomenon has long been studied in terms of development, findings that are more recent illustrate plasticity of the brain throughout the life span. That is, people can learn at any stage in life and the brain will continue to reorganize to accommodate said learning (Bruer, 1998). The underlying assumption behind life-long learning and neuroplasticity for leadership practice is the notion that if the optimal brain-functioning patterns for leaders can be identified, those patterns of functioning can be elicited in, and subsequently learned by, organizational leaders to improve their effectiveness.

Researchers have begun to explore the usefulness of neuroscience on improvement of leadership skills is through neurofeedback. Neurofeedback entails connecting the subject to a neurological monitoring device, such as an EEG (electroencephalograph), and measuring their brain activity while performing certain tasks. By providing the participants with constant feedback, they are able to optimally tune their neurological functioning during the task. Neurofeedback has been used successfully in treating various cognitive disorders, for conditioning athletes, and for relieving stress. It has also been suggested for use within the organizational science domain to help leaders develop and improve psychological capital (Peterson, Waldman, Balthazard, & Thatcher, 2008) by facilitating successful interaction skills. Leaders with high degrees of psychological capital are thought to be more effective, and it is suggested that neurofeedback and coaching may help leaders to improve upon individual components of psychological capital, such as resiliency or confidence (Peterson et al., 2008).

While the idea of potentially using neuroscience information and practice to improve an individual's level of leadership skill is intriguing, and merits investigation, we must consider several questions that appear not to have been raised as yet. First, studies such as Peterson et al. (2008) compare different brain patterns across individuals to identify high and low degrees of skill acquisition. As noted earlier, simply identifying a region of brain activation only correlates it with a given skill set, and does not represent any degree of causality of differential functioning. Certainly, other individual differences in brain functioning must be considered, especially in light of the fact that neuroplasticity exists and the brain can adapt. As such, differential levels of activation across individuals do not necessarily indicate different levels of skill.

Additionally, we have examined, largely due to cost constraints, a limited subject pool consisting of individuals already functioning as leaders. Clearly, this presents an issue of range restriction that limits the extent to which conclusions may be drawn or results generalized. Additionally, it remains unknown whether the effects of training methods, such as neurofeedback, are temporally stable. In the absence of such evidence, organizations could possibly spend large amounts of money on research and practice, the effects of which are ultimately diminished before they can even be put to use.

A cross-disciplinary examination of the application of neuroscience within other domains sheds some light on additional concerns that are of immediate consequence to its application within the leadership domain. Lessons can be learned, for example, by reviewing attempts made to incorporate neuroscience research into educational practices. Alferink and Farmer-Dougan (2010) examine several primary issues with the relationship previously forged between neuroscience and education. The first criticism highlighted surrounds misinterpretations of research on brain lateralization that has led to the development of inappropriate teaching strategies. Brain lateralization refers to the fact that the human brain is comprised of two distinct hemispheres that are joined in the middle by the corpus callosum. Lateralization may be thought of as a broad form of localization. It is widely accepted that each hemisphere is responsible for differential processing of information, and education curricula have been developed to allow instructors to teach to specific hemispheres.

For example, researchers have posited that the left side of the brain is responsible for logical information processing while the right side of the brain is responsible for spatial pattern recognition and creativity. Education curricula are designed for both hemispheres in an effort to deliver information in ways targeting an individual's strengths, or in a remedial case, to compensate for perceived brain-based weaknesses. While intuitively appealing, the changes in teaching curricula rooted in these neuroscientific discoveries are based upon partial truths and misunderstandings. The reality is that information, although processed different by each hemisphere, is also processed simultaneously by each hemisphere. Therefore, the hemispherical targeted educational tools developed are not being processed by any one given hemisphere, yielding spurious conclusions. In addition, it is unclear as to whether or not the learner stands to benefit by not integrating information across hemispheres (Alferink & Farmer-Dougan, 2010).

Another criticism by Alferink and Farmer-Dougan (2010) surrounds the misunderstanding of neurological development. Whereas it is widely understood and accepted that the brain and neurological system undergo a reliable pattern of change associated with human growth and development, the outcomes of these changes are not as widely accepted. For example, it is unclear as to whether or not an optimal period in the developmental cycle exists for learning. Instead, it is more likely that different types of learning are more successful at different developmental periods. However, based on accepted developmental information, educators have decided that learning develops the most and fastest at early developmental stages, leaving children better able to learn than adults. Alferink and Farmer-Dougan (2010) highlight issues with the popular notion of teaching to a "learning style," one that has developed through the union of neuroscience and education research. It is widely believed that we possess different forms of intelligence (Gardner, 1983) and that individual learning is best accomplished by teaching to a style, or modality, that is congruent with the individual's intelligence profile (Sprenger, 1999).

Unfortunately, research findings do not support this popular notion, and it is likely that overly focusing education toward one modality will limit an individual's ability to use alternate modalities (Alferink & Farmer-Dougan, 2010). Clearly, the more tools one has at one's disposal, the more effective he or she can be across a variety of situations. Putting "all your eggs in one basket" is likely not a good educational strategy, organizational strategy, or leadership strategy. In fact, cognitive research has demonstrated that global commands (such as those that operate both hands) are likely the default for neural connections, and the execution of finely tuned commands (such as operate the left hand only) requires overriding the default. Thus, it is now believed that the neurological system operates in a far more integrated fashion than originally expected (Diamond, 2009). In that light, attempts to teach to specific modalities or to promote specific psychological capacities believed to increase leadership skills may be less useful than expected.

Alferink and Farmer-Dougan (2010) go on to highlight additional issues such as over-interpreting data, measurement error, and validity concerns similar to those already discussed. They conclude that, at best, neuroscientific research may support current education practices, but it does not appear to improve them at all. In considering how to apply neuroscience to leadership, similar concerns exist. Certainly, we do not want to advocate the training of individual leadership styles (akin to modalities) at the expense of others. The contextual component of effective leadership practice is well known (Van Vugt, Hogan, & Kaiser, 2008). Likewise, we do not want to invest organizational resources in developing curricula based on information that is not fully understood, such as the curriculum established surrounding brain lateralization.

Unfortunately, current directions in neuroscience (i.e., localization) appear to be propelling us towards similar problems if carried into an applied setting. If neuroscience has only supported existing education policies but not improved upon them (Alferink & Farmer-Dougan, 2010), where is the utility for organizations when we meet these same conclusions in years to come? Questions/concerns may well find answers through continued research. However, we must be prudent in the degree to which we allow the integration of neuroscience into the leadership domain. History suggests a pattern of moving forward too quickly and not fully developing and understanding what neuroscience does and does not have to offer.

As organizational scientists, we must be prudent to avoid the same premature integration. Researchers in education continue to call for prudence in applying neurological evidence to guide practice (Wolfe & Brandt, 1998). It would appear that once the cat got out of the bag, scientists in the educational domain have been hard pressed to stave off a knowledge-thirsty public willing to accept informational inaccuracies due to their mass appeal. Unfortunately, this phenomenon is not limited to the educational domain. Early pioneers in neurological research have reflected on the misuse of their work by the public and expressed concern that the introduction of neuroscience to organizational science may meet with a similar fate (Dvorak & Badal, 2007).

OTHER BIOLOGICAL APPROACHES TO UNDERSTANDING LEADERSHIP

Neuroscience represents one particularly alluring avenue toward a biology of leadership; however, there are other biological approaches, specifically physiological approaches that should also be considered. Indeed, physiological measures have been employed within the organizational research domain for some time, as evident from Wright and Diamond's (2006) historical account of the use of cardiovascular measurement in examining employee behaviors. Thus, a discussion of leadership from a biological perspective should include considerations from more "classic" physiological domains, as well as modern neuroscientific approaches.

Physiological studies have a historical and increasingly close tie to organizational sciences, primarily in the study of job stress (Cooper, Dewe, & O'Driscoll, 2001). In borrowing from job stress literature, elements of concern arise that must be taken into account when subsequently pairing biological factors with leadership. Of primary concern in examining physiological measurement within the organizational science domain is measurement error.

Physiological measurement can provide a wealth of information, yet the meaning of this information is frequently subject to misinterpretation due to the limited understanding of these phenomena. One depiction of this challenge can be found in Wright and Diamond's (2006) account of the historical use of cardiovascular measures (specifically, pulse rate, systolic and diastolic blood pressure). The study revealed a decades-long learning curve in the evolving interpretation of these early measures. Particularly puzzling to early organizational researchers was the finding that pulse rate and systolic pressure (SBP) positively correlated with workload, whereas diastolic pressure (DBP) was negatively related. Ultimately, findings suggested a composite cardiovascular measure was most appropriate, yet even at the tail end of the curve, organizational researchers and practitioners attempting to connect chronic heart disease (CHD) with job stress and age continued to misinterpret cardiovascular measures (Wright & Diamond, 2006). From this historical perspective, traditional risk factors for CHD were determined from systolic and diastolic blood pressure measurement (Wright & Diamond, 2006).

It was not until 1999, as part of the longitudinal Framingham Heart Study, that researchers (Franklin, Khan, Wong, Larson, & Levy, 1999) revealed that traditional interpretations of blood pressure alone (SBP & DBP) were not accurate and likely to be dangerously misleading. A composite measure of blood pressure, known as pulse pressure (PP), was determined to be the best predictor of CHD risk over SBP and DBP alone. Pulse pressure is the difference score between systolic and diastolic pressures. Specific findings showed CHD risk was positively associated with SBP, DBP, and PP when the variables were examined individually. This appeared contrary to the traditional belief that CHD risk was negatively associated with DBP. However, when examined together, SBP showed a positive association with CHD and DBP showed a negative association. These findings are more consistent with traditional beliefs. This contradiction again demonstrates the ease of misinterpretation and the potential learning curve that is required when examining recently recognized physiological phenomenon. Ultimately, Franklin et al. (1999) suggested that PP is a key component in examining risk factors for CHD and is able to account for individual differences in relationships between SBP and DBP that appear to confuse researchers when examining the predictive nature of SPB and DBP on CHD.

The illustration of this learning curve demonstrates our current, limited understanding of the physiological measures used in organizational research today. Work stress researchers have explored many physiological measures including heart rate and salivary cortisol (Lac & Chamoux, 2004);

salivary cortisol and urinary catecholamine (Fujigaki & Mori, 1997); blood serum lipids (high/low density lipoproteins or cholesterol) and fibrinogens (Bernin, Theorell, & Sandberg, 2001); blood glucose levels, prolactin, testosterone, and cortisol (Grossi, Theorell, Jürisoo, & Setterlind, 1999); urinary epinephrine and norepinephrine (catecholamine), and cortisol (Evans & Johnson, 2000); urinary epinephrine and norepinephrine, catecholimines, and blood pressure (Melin, Lundberg, Söderlund, & Granqvist, 1999); and serum cholesterol, uric acid, serum triglycerides, and systolic/diastolic blood pressure (Steffy & Jones, 1988).

Although this list is meant to be representative and not exhaustive, it highlights the fact that identifying reliable relationships between physiological indicators and job stress is still very much a work in progress. Further exploration into the findings connecting physiological indicators and job stress reveals a limited understanding of the interpretation of these measures or what these measures indicate. In fact, the evidence is often contradictory. For example, Evans and Johnson (2000) concluded that elevated epinephrine levels were a reliable indicator of stress, elevated norepinephrine levels indicated physical exertion, and cortisol changes were associated with psychological distress. However, Hansen, Kaergaard, Anderson, and Netterstroms (2003) found differences in catabolic (plasma HbA1c) and anabolic (testosterone) hormonal levels between groups performing repetitive tasks (typically associated with job stress) and groups performing non-repetitive work, but found no between-group differences for other physiological markers including cortisol, epinephrine, and norepinephrine.

Similarly, Bernin et al. (2001) found blood serum lipids (i.e., cholesterol) to be most strongly related to corporate psychosocial factors (corporate culture), and cortisol levels to be an indicator of arousal (may be due to either beneficial or detrimental circumstances). In a study of academics, Bekker, de Jong, Zijlstra, and van Landeghem (2000) reported no differences in cortisol levels between high stress, dual-role participants (those with children and careers) and lower stress, single-role (career only) participants, whereas Lac and Chamoux (2004) reported significant differences in cortisol levels between high- and lower-stress groups of factory workers. These contradictory findings illuminate the quagmire of combinations of physiological measures and work stress and the equivocal nature of the results. For example, cortisol is shown to be both related and unrelated to work stress—not a very probative conclusion.

In reviewing the work stress literature, it is clear that the current understanding and interpretation of complex physiological measures is, at best, equivocal. While the findings of some studies have been consistent with one another, the findings of other studies have directly contradicted one another. Seemingly, this would allow for numerous Type I (false positives), Type II (false negatives), and Type III (correctly rejecting the null hypothesis but for the wrong reason) errors in this research stream. Although our understanding of blood pressure and pulse rate reactions has evolved historically (Wright & Diamond, 2006), the current understanding of other measures appears best represented by the often divergent conclusions reached by researchers in those fields. What is necessary, before reliable conclusions can be drawn based on physiological measurement, is a more thorough understanding of what the measures reveal, how they interact with one another, and agreement and replication across multiple studies. Until then, organizational researchers must be cautious in drawing any conclusions concerning work stress or leadership based on biological evidence.

Researchers have yet to address the inconsistencies that appear throughout the work stress literature. As seen in the decades-long progression of understanding blood pressure measures (Wright & Diamond, 2006), limited understanding of complex physiological measures has led to confusion and misinterpretation of findings. It is critical that the research community work to solidify a complete and thorough understanding of variables of interest prior to drawing conclusions based on their measurement. This can only be achieved through continued study of accepted measures and successful replication of obtained results. For organizational sciences, measures must be agreed upon, well defined, and fully operationalized. Only then can studies be replicated, results be accepted, and potentially generalizable conclusions be drawn.

In the current state, multiple physiological measures are examined for the same construct, with little (if any) replication across studies and widespread equivocal (if not contradictory) results. Furthermore, in some research, physiological measures are viewed as outcome variables and sometimes they are viewed as predictor variables, and in a number of instances, research has failed to separate these instances. These issues must be resolved before considering the place of human physiological measurement in organizational science, and should serve as a valuable cautionary flag when considering the pairing of neuroscience and leadership. The issues that remain present in applying physiological measurement to organizational sciences are parallel to those faced by the application of neuroscience to leadership. In the former research stream, proceeding too quickly and an apparent lack of addressing these concerns has led to an extant literature fraught with contradictions and confusion. Early caution and prudence on the part of the research community can prevent repeating history's mistakes in this case.

LIVING HAPPILY EVER AFTER: CAN PHYSIOLOGY ANSWER THE QUESTIONS THAT WILL MOVE LEADERSHIP RESEARCH FORWARD?

Up to this point, we have suggested a number of the shortcomings associated with investigating psychological phenomena with physiologically-based methods. Provided that these limitations are confronted and addressed, it is important to consider what the increased use of physiological measurement in leadership research can tell us about the leadership process. For instance, neuroscience has the potential to identify which areas of the brain are activated when psychological phenomena occur. However, as Burge (2010) points out, "Correlations between localized neural activity and specific psychological phenomena are important facts. But they merely set the stage for explanation. Being purely descriptive, they explain nothing." Thus, in this section we look at the field of leadership's most pressing leadership needs over both the past ten years and the next ten years in order to gauge the prudence of a shift of our limited scholarly resources toward the study of physiology in leadership.

Recently, Gardner, Lowe, Moss, Mahoney, and Cogliser (2010) reviewed the last ten years of the journal's work, and provided a set of research directions for leadership researchers in the next decade. In short, their recommendations center on moving away from retrospective survey-based research toward more insightful and creative, yet equally if not more valid, measures of leadership behavior. Indeed, the authors encourage the increased use of lab studies, quasi-experimental studies, content analyses, multi-study projects, public opinion polls, cross-level studies, and so forth. Although diverse, all of these methods are heavily utilized and well-validated by many other branches of the organizational sciences. Prudently, these authors are shining a light on some of the methods that leadership scholars have, to a large extent, raced by in the rapid expansion of leadership research over the past two decades.

That is not to say that leadership researchers should not interact with other disciplines outside of organizational research. Once again Gardner et al. (2010) point out that sociologists, behavioral economists, and even cognitive scientists can bring rich perspectives and techniques to the study of leadership in organizations. The caveat here is that these disciplines have an extensive set of highly valid methods with which they conduct their research. It appears that Gardner and colleagues are encouraging leadership researchers to tap into these methods and reap the innovative findings that they might generate.

With all of the highly valid and well-used methods, both within organizational research and outside of it, that hold great potential for unlocking some of leadership's mysteries, it begs the question of why resources should be spent on still-developing methods based in neuroscience or other physiological measurement. This is not a question of whether some insights can be gleaned from these techniques—clearly they can. It is a question of whether an investment of scholarly resources into physiology by leadership scholars is productive at this point. To gain further support for our contention that the answer to this question is "not yet," we also took a look at a previous attempt at developing suggestions to move leadership research forward.

A decade prior, Lowe and Gardner (2000) identified several areas for future research in leadership studies to demonstrate how future leadership work can most contribute to practitioner needs and scholarly knowledge in the 21st century. Again, we briefly explore each area and consider the potential contribution of physiologically based methods compared against the more traditional methods, many of which, such as longitudinal, qualitative, and quasi-experimental designs, are already not used frequently enough. As we will argue, in most cases, the finite supply of leadership research resources may be better spent on investigating leadership phenomena through these highly valid and more intensive approaches instead of the trendier, yet less valid physiological measures.

First, further research is needed on the relationship between top management groups and strategic leadership and decision making (Lowe & Gardner, 2000). While much progress has been made over the past decade concerning top management team processes (Carpenter, Geletkanycz, & Sanders, 2004), there is still much work to be done to approach the level of understanding of decision making at this level of the organization that we possess at the employee-level of the organization. The reason for this, beyond the nascent nature of this stream of research, is not lack of proper methods, but lack of access to leaders at this level on which to practice our existing methods. Thus, while physiological study may give us some insight into top level decision making, our traditional methods, especially longitudinal and qualitative work, have yet to be applied deeply enough to glean the deep, rich insights that these methods provide. On a more practical note, we can only speculate that, as difficult as it is to get top management teams to fill out surveys, it will be eminently more challenging to gain their consent for brain scans, cortisol spit samples, or blood pressure checks—almost anything that requires hooking up to a piece of machinery.

Next, Lowe and Gardner (2000) suggested that future leadership research should test existing theory at multiple levels of analysis. Indeed, this is a common plea from many areas of the organizational sciences. Over the past decade, methodologists and statisticians have continued to provide researchers with an array of newer tools and techniques, such as hierarchical linear modeling, for studying and analyzing organizational phenomena at multiple levels of analysis. Physiological measures, by their nature, seem best suited to operate at the individual level. While, of course, individual measurements of brain activity could be aggregated to the team or organization level, interpreting the precise meaning of this higher-level variable appears fraught with both difficulty and uncertainly.

The process through which leadership systems develop leadership knowledge, skills, and abilities is another fruitful area for future research (Lowe & Gardner, 2000). While this seems on the surface to be an area where physiological measurement may help explain changes in development over time, we have already pointed out, in our discussion of neurofeedback, that this method may not yet be sophisticated enough to capture individual growth over time. Further, relatively little work in leadership thus far has combined existing measures of leadership with more advanced methodological tools for modeling change over time such as latent growth models and random coefficient modeling (Ployhart & Vandenberg, 2010). This suggests that lack of measures is not the primary constraint to this of research; instead, the challenge of collecting measures of leader attitudes and behavior over time appears to be the more pressing and important challenge. Thus, while physiological measures may be of value to the study of leadership development at some point in the future, that time does not seem to have arrived.

Lowe and Gardner (2000) also recommend that future work be conducted that examines how context influences leader attitudes, emotions, and behavior. For example, international settings, social networks, technological changes, and political climates may all impact how managers lead a successful organization and its employees. Here again, physiological measures do not seem to have a noteworthy advantage over traditional measures. As in many of these areas for future research, physiology may provide a useful secondary source of reliability in these contexts, but due to its aforementioned limitations, we caution against even that at this point.

Further, as Lowe and Gardner (2000) pointed out, the subject of women as leaders continues to be a significant area of study for leadership researchers as well as practicing human resource professionals. Here, physiological measures may indeed provide meaningful explanatory power in exploring the differences in attitudes and emotions between female and male leaders. However, the groundwork of psychological differences between men and women, as measured by physiological indicators, is still being developed by competent researchers in psychology and neuroscience.

Therefore, we question the wisdom of spending a large amount of resources pursuing these differences before these "mother disciplines" of the psychology–physiology link do. Perhaps a more prudent approach would be to wait until these other disciplines conduct more foundational work in detecting psychological differences in gender via physiology before proceeding with our own. This way, not only will the measures be more refined at this later stage, but these leadership and gender studies can be developed by generalizing the findings from other disciplines, thereby resulting in more theoretically grounded advances.

In sum, we recognize that the use of physiological measures to study psychological phenomena in organizational research may be useful in some areas. Indeed, Akinola (2010) suggests that the areas of affect, trust, power, conflict, diversity, and health may all be ripe for the use of this new methodological technology. Clearly, like nearly all organizational phenomena, these areas intersect with leadership in a number of ways. However, as we have argued, significant benefits for our understanding of what scholars consider the most pressing areas for future leadership study are not apparent. When this contention is combined with the previously discussed validity-based shortcomings of these measures, we begin to get cold feet concerning the marriage of leadership psychology and physiology.

CONCLUSION

Does the bundling and marriage of neuroscience and leadership end happily ever after? The answer seems as unclear as attempting to predict the success of any marriage in today's world. What does appear clear is that the domain of neuroscience has some growing pains, development, and fine-tuning of its own to work out. Researchers within that field continue to call for consistency across methodologies and analyses (Kriegeskorte et al., 2009; Vul et al., 2009; Kriegeskorte et al., 2010). Until such milestones are reached, results and subsequent conclusions drawn from neurological research should be viewed through a cautionary lens that highlights the threats to validity currently hampering the domain. Other disciplines (including organizational sciences and leadership) should be wary of the degree to which they allow themselves to mingle with neuroscience, in its present state.

The high-stakes environment informed by organizational science and leadership studies makes us even more cautious. As Berridge (2004) suggested, and as we have argued in relation to leadership, there are many factors more important in understanding human behavior that neuroscience, due to the weak practical implications of neuroscience research. Understanding the relationships that result in set shifting and visual attention seems to us to be quite a long way removed from what happens in the leadership process. Furthermore, Messick's (1996) idea of consequential evidence for construct validity suggests that the consequences of psychological measurement are an integral part of what is commonly known as construct validity.

It is our duty, as researchers, to guard our field and the consumers of our knowledge (organizations and their leaders) against the consequences of misinterpreting research findings or misguiding practice based on research lacking in validity. Kagan (2007) notes that whereas experts within each field (i.e., neuroscience) are not likely to misinterpret findings (e.g., any activation of the amygdala signals a heightened fear response), this may not be the case for researchers in other fields or the public. Misinterpretation of experimental findings (either by the researcher or reader) leading to incorrect action in an applied setting should be considered a threat to construct validity by virtue of consequence, and must be guarded against.

Weisberg et al. (2008) compared levels of satisfaction with explanation of psychological phenomena across conditions (good/bad explanation, and with/without neuroscience information) and across groups (novices selected from the general public, neuroscience students, and neuroscience experts). Their findings indicated individuals from all groups were generally more satisfied with good explanations of psychological phenomena and those that included neuroscience information. The most interesting result, however, was that novices from the general public were fairly satisfied with bad explanations that contained neuroscience information and not at all satisfied with bad explanations that did not contain any neuroscience information. These results were true of the student sample as well; only the neuroscience subject matter experts displayed dissatisfaction with bad explanations that also included neuroscience information. Not all readers are expert, and whether due to their limited knowledge of a particular field or the heightened influence of scientific exploration that happens to be intriguing and popularized by increased attention from the scientific community, it is clear that some may be easily misled.

The Weisberg et al. (2008) study empirically demonstrates Kagan's (2007) earlier cautions, which should not be limited to researchers within neuroscience. As organizational scientists, readers from many disciplines are attentive to our work. Many of them are practicing professionals who rely on us as subject matter experts, and we must be diligent in our understanding of neuroscience and presentation of neuroscientific evidence, or risk misleading readers, organizations, leaders, and even the general public (Weisberg, 2008). The misuse of neuroscientific evidence may result in incorrect conclusions with serious consequences (beyond a scathing critique by a journal editor or peer) when findings are implemented within an organization, or used to guide policy and decision-making within organization life. As such, Messick's (1996) idea of consequence as evidence of validity should be carefully considered as we seek a relationship between neuroscience and leadership.

Directly resulting from our highlighted concerns surrounding methodological and analytical shortcomings, and the potential for unwelcome (or at least misguided) consequences, it is our feeling that the bundling and marriage of neuroscience and leadership, at least for now, is likely more problematic than productive. We must make it clear—we are NOT neuroscientists but we must also make it clear that we have come to this conclusion in our roles as the modal readership of the organizational science/ leadership literature. In that role, we echo the call of fellow researchers that have implored caution and pause before jumping on the neuroscience bandwagon (Dvorak & Badal, 2007; Wolfe & Brandt, 1998). At the same time, working toward a biology of leadership may likely be a welcome addition to the leadership research stream, assuming it is developed with proper scientific rigor.

Perhaps a longer period of supervised courting before marriage, or the erection of a large bundling board to keep the areas from intimately intertwining, is the most prudent course of action before deciding the future of neuroscience and leadership research. We implore our colleagues using the same phrase that American football analyst Lee Corso frequently exclaims to his fellow football prognosticators when he feels they are not taking into account all relevant and available information while determining their prediction of the victor of a soon-to-be-played game: "Not so fast, my friend!"

NOTE

We appreciate the comments of Gerald R. Ferris and Pamela L. Perrewé on an earlier version of this manuscript. Address correspondence to: M. Ronald Buckley, University of Oklahoma, Division of Management, Norman, OK 73019, E-mail: mbuckley@ou.edu

REFERENCES

Akinola, M. (2010). Measuring the pulse of an organization: Integrating physiological measures into the organizational scholar's toolbox. *Research in Organizational Behavior, 30*, 203–223.

Alferink, L.A., & Farmer-Dougan, V. (2010). Brain-(not) based education: Dangers of misunderstanding and misapplication of neuroscience research. *Exceptionality, 18*, 42–52.

Bekker, M. H. J., de Jong, P. F., Zijlstra, F. R. H., & van Landeghem, B.A.J. (2000). Combining care and work: Health and stress effects in male and female academics. *International Journal of Behavioral Medicine, 7*, 28–43.

Bernin, P., Theorell, T., & Sandberg, C.G. (2001). Biological correlates of social support and pressure at work in managers. *Integrative Physiological and Behavioral Science, 36*, 121–136.

Berridge K.C. (2004). Motivation concepts in behavioral neuroscience. *Physiology and Behaviour, 81*,179–209.

Bruer, J.T. (1998). Brain science, brain fiction. *Educational Leadership, 56,* 14–18.

Burge, T. (2010, December 19). A real science of the mind. *The New York Times.* Retrieved from http://opinionator.blogs.nytimes.com/2010/12/19/a-real-science-of-mind/

Cacioppo, J.T., Lorig, T.S., Berntson, G.G., Norris, C.J., Rickett, E., & Nusbaum, H. (2003). Just because you're imaging the brain doesn't mean you can stop using your head: A primer and set of first principles. *Journal of Personality and Social Psychology, 85,* 650–661.

Carpenter, M.A., Geletkanycz, M.A., & Sanders, W.G. (2004). Upper echelons research revisited: Antecedents, elements, and consequences of top management team composition. *Journal of Management, 30,* 749–778.

Cooper, C.L., Dewe, P.J., & O'Driscoll, M.P. (2001). *Organizational stress: A review and critique of theory, research, and applications.* Thousand Oaks, CA: Sage.

Diamond, A. (2009). All or none hypothesis: A global-default mode that characterizes the brain and mind. *Developmental Psychology, 45,* 130–138.

Dvorak, P., & Badal, J. (2007, September 20). This is your brain on the job—Neuroscientists are finding that business leaders really may think differently. *The Wall Street Journal,* B1.

Evans, G.W., & Johnson, D. (2000). Stress and open-office noise. *Journal of Applied Psychology, 85,* 779–783.

Franklin, S.S., Khan, S.A., Wong, N.D., Larson, M.G., & Levy, D. (1999). Is pulse pressure useful in predicting risk for coronary heart disease? The Framingham heart study. *Circulation, 100,* 354–360.

Fujigaki, Y., & Mori, K. (1997). Longitudinal study of work stress among information system professional. *International Journal of Human-Computer Interaction, 9,* 369–381.

Gardner, H. (1983). *Frames of mind: The theory of multiple intelligences.* New York, NY: Basic Books.

Gardner, W.L., Lowe, K.B., Moss, T.W., Mahoney, K.T., & Cogliser, C.C. (2010). Scholarly leadership of the study of leadership: A review of *The Leadership Quarterly*'s second decade, 2000–2009. *Leadership Quarterly, 21,* 922–958.

Grossi, G., Theorell, T., Jürisoo, M., & Setterlind, S. (1999). Psychophysiological correlates of organizational change and threat of unemployment among police inspectors. *Integrative Physiological and Behavioral Science, 34,* 30–42.

Hansen, A.M., Kaergaard, A., Andersen, J.H., & Netterstroms, B. (2003). Association between repetitive work and endocrinological indicators of stress. *Work & Stress, 17,* 264–276.

Kagan, J. (2007). A trio of concerns. *Perspectives on Psychological Science, 2,* 361–376.

Kriegeskorte, N., Simmons, W.K., Bellgowan, P.S.F., & Bake, C.I. (2009). Circular analysis in systems neuroscience—The dangers of double dipping. *Nature Neuroscience, 12,* 535–540.

Kriegeskorte, N., Lindquist, M.A., Nichols, T.E., Poldrack, R.A., & Vul, E. (2010). Everything you never wanted to know about circular analysis, but were afraid to ask. *Journal of Cerebral Blood Flow & Metabolism, 30,* 1–7.

Lac, G., & Chamoux, A. (2004). Biological and psychological responses to two rapid shiftwork schedules. *Ergonomics, 47,* 1339–1349.

Lederhendler, I., & Schulkin, J. (2000). Behavioral neuroscience: Challenges for the era of molecular biology. *Trends in Neuroscience, 23*, 451–454.

Lowe, K.B., & Gardner, W.L. (2000). Ten years of *The Leadership Quarterly*: Contributions and challenges for the future. *The Leadership Quarterly, 11*, 459–514.

Melin, B.O., Lundberg, U., Söderlund, J., & Granqvist, M. (1999). Psychological and physiological stress reaction of male and female assembly workers: A comparison between two different forms of work organization. *Journal of Organizational Behavior, 20*, 47–61.

Messick, S. (1996). Validity of psychological assessment: Validation inferences from persons' responses and performance as scientific inquiry into score meaning. *American Psychologist, 50*, 741–749.

Petersen, s. J., Waldman, D. A., Balthazard, P. A., & Thatcher, R. W. (2008). Neuroscientific applications of psychological capital: Are the brains of optimistic, hopeful, confident, and resilient leaders different? *Organizational Dynamics, 37*(4), 342–353.

Ployhart, R.E., & Vandenberg, R.J. (2010). Longitudinal research: The theory, design, and analysis of change. *Journal of Management, 36*, 94–120.

Ringleb, A.H., & Rock, D. (2008). The emerging field of neuroleadership. *Neuroleadership Journal, 1*, 1–17.

Sprenger, M. (1999). *Learning and memory: The brain in action.* Alexandria, VA: Association for Supervision and Curriculum Development.

Steffy, B., & Jones, J. (1988). Workplace stress and indicators of coronary-disease risk. *Academy of Management Journal, 31*, 686–698.

Van Vugt, M., Hogan, R., & Kaiser, R.B. (2008). Leadership, followership, and evolution: Some lessons from the past. *American Psychologist, 63*, 182–196.

Vul, E., Harris, C., Winkielman, P., & Pashler, H. (2009). Puzzingly high correlations in fMRI studies of emotion, personality, and social cognition. *Perspectives on Psychological Science, 4*, 274–290.

Weisberg, D.S. (2008). Caveat lector: The presentation of neuroscience information in the popular media. *The Scientific Review of Mental Health Practices, 6*, 51–56.

Weisberg, D.S., Keil, F.C., Goodstein, J., Rawson, E., & Gray, J.R. (2008). The seductive allure of neuroscience explanations. *Journal of Cognitive Neuroscience, 20*, 470–477.

White, R. E., Thornhill, S., & Hampson, E. (2007). A biosocial model of entrepreneurship: The combined effects of nurture and nature. *Journal of Organizational Behavior, 28*, 451–466.

Wolfe, P., & Brandt, R. (1998). What do we know from brain research? *Educational Leadership*, 8–13.

Wright, T.A., & Diamond, J.W. (2006). Getting the 'pulse' of your employees: The use of cardiovascular research in better understanding behavior in organizations. *Journal of Organizational Behavior, 27*, 395–401.

CHAPTER 12

PEOPLE MANAGEMENT

A Psychosomatic View and Commentary

Artur Zular

Businesses, organizations with a very long history, reinvent themselves day by day. Consisting of people, businesses, with their conflictive relationships, are playing an increasingly important role in people's lives. Up to a short time ago, this role belonged to the family. Even if they do not wish to do so, modern women and men spend more and more of their time at work in the business and for the business. When they are not there, they are either coming from it or going to it, and the time spent in transit has steadily increased. Much of the little time left for home is taken up by thinking of business-related problems, whether answering e-mails or writing reports and presentations.

So even though it may go unnoticed, family relations, life outside work, leisure, sports, hobbies, charity activities, and friends ultimately receive less attention because of absolute lack of time. On other occasions, the problem is not lack of time, but the individual who, contaminated by the current practice, ends up prioritizing the firm, at the expense of an appropriate balance in all spheres of life.

Coping and Prevention, pages 219–229

Directors of today's companies, I would not dare say modern companies, repeat mistakes and faults of the past, which are transmitted with the strength and determination of a gene in a hereditary disease.

The person who becomes a boss, in most cases, is not trained for it. Generally it is the employee who has been longest with the firm, is more experienced, or else someone brought in from the competition. In the former case, promotion is a prize that comes in the form of a raise in salary and better benefits, progress in a career path scheme, in case there is one, and higher social status. The new boss now begins to give orders as he used to be given, and make demands, as used to be made of him. He replicates what has always happened and, consciously or unconsciously, he has a guarantee that everything will work out. But from this point of view, the fact that it works does not mean that it is the most appropriate way of doing things. Reproducing a modus operandi makes sure that the product will be produced, that goods will be sold, or that services will be provided. But what about quality? At what price, both material and human? At this point the relationship of the individual versus productivity speaks louder.

For some time now the corporate market has realized the pressing need to invest in people management. A lot is heard about training methods referring to high performance, motivation, leadership, empowerment, and many others, offered as fast food snacks. This Manichean view of training and capacity-building that currently prevails among us generates products as though they were meant for rats subjected to Pavlovian conditioning. But unlike guinea pigs that can repeat a movement endless times on hearing a bell, human beings feel and think, and they interpret their feelings and create positive and negative affects towards all and any events in their life. Were this not enough, they have affective memory, that is, something in the present that, unconsciously, makes them establish an association with a positive or negative past experience, may make the present feeling seem strange but consistent with what they experienced in the past.

Human beings, like any animal, have instincts, but unlike animals that only rely on instincts to determine their survival through a relationship, mating and perpetuation of the species, human beings have an extremely gifted psychological apparatus. Through reason, human beings make choices through a dynamic balance between instinct and rationality that results in more or less spontaneous actions, gestures, and behaviors that are more or less adapted to a specific situation and time.

During pregnancy, all the child's organs and systems are prepared by an incredible cell differentiation process. When it is born, its tiny organs are formed and relate to each other like well-tuned instruments of a philharmonic orchestra without the presence of a conductor.

The cardiovascular system is ready and, although minuscule, at this time the heart has all the predetermined functions taking place in perfect tune with veins, arteries, and lungs. The respiratory system, which was immersed in the amniotic fluid, suddenly begins to have air that fills the bronchi and pulmonary alveoli that will take oxygen to the blood. The blood is already there and it will be pumped by the little heart that is already born beating at a steady pace. The same occurs with the gastrointestinal system, skeletal muscles, and genitourinary system. Some functions will need time to improve; others will take years to be structured, such as fertility, but there they are, waiting for their inexorable fate. The only exception, that is, the only system that is not born with a person and depends on external operators to be installed—"managers and bosses"—is the psychological apparatus.

The human mind is formed by influxes that are experienced during the first eight years of life, which we call the forming phase. This forming depends on the person and on what form these experiences will take place. Logically there is a genetic material that in some way predisposes to certain behaviors, but it is the interaction with mother and father, or with equivalent parental figures such as uncles and aunts, grandparents, servants or even the educators in an orphanage, that will determine how the individual's psychological apparatus will be. To this interaction is added the relationship with other family members, friends, teachers, directors, church, and customs and laws of different societies and cultures in the process of psychological differentiation and mental development. This constellation of factors is responsible for the fact that no two people on the face of the earth are the same. Even if they are identical or monozygotic twins, that is, from the same cell—same egg and sperm—they will have different experiences, even if similar ones, since the input and psychological processing will be different.

In companies, there are bosses who think that whatever they want to happen will happen. Because it worked with so-and-so, it will now work with someone else. Because they did it this way at the other company, the same will happen at this one. However, each individual is unique or, as they say, "each to his own way."

The same script played by different actors creates the show of life as a novelesque comedy or a Shakespearean tragedy. Each actor on the business scene has his or her own history and a particular culture that, when introjected over the course of life, outlines behavioral patterns that are very difficult to change. Understanding and assimilating these processes does not take place in a uniform manner because of these factors, and not knowing this has cost the businesses very dearly.

In the corporate world, bosses are changed like soccer team coaches. When they are hired, for a huge amount of money, it is because the club leaders want the coach to now repeat the success achieved the previous season with the other team. But at this point in time, this is another team, with different experiences, different skills, other insecurities, other fears, other limitations. When they do not manage to reproduce the incredible victories, nor live up to the expectations of those who hired them, they frustrate the hiring party's expectations and are soon fired. What happened? Was this coach who was so highly praised, with an exceptional résumé and appreciated for his results, actually not as good and as competent as expected? Or was it the team of players that was actually not as talented as the other team? Possibly the answer is neither one nor the other. Teams are groups of talented people who have to present results through their individual competencies and their capacity to get along as a team, and they have to constantly interpret the changes going on in their field of action. There is a great expectation for results and the quality of the work done is checked at the same time by thousands of analysts—the fans—working as a real-time audit. In another situation, a marvelous soccer player will not always become a competent coach. As we said previously, promoting an excellent and more experienced coworker to a managerial position does not guarantee that we will have a competent boss. The result may be that he is a mediocre boss. Referring to soccer, once again, the recent Brazilian record in the World Cup showed precisely this.

People management is definitely more complicated than it seems. It is easy to give orders, but leading people properly, while respecting the difficulty inherent in the task, requires knowledge, intelligence, and wisdom. What is unique about Psychosomatic People Management is the fact that it analyzes the process from the biopsychosocial standpoint. If, on the one hand, the coworker is a unique being and makes that particular company unique, on the other hand, he is a biological being, with a differentiated psychological system and a complicated web of social relations.

Most reports on productivity problems are related to the lack of team motivation. Essentially, this is caused by the difficulty in understanding how to deal with that group of people. Try to serve, at a very fine restaurant, a marvelous, juicy tenderloin dish to a vegetarian. Regardless of its price, of the effort that went into its preparation, the careful presentation, the cook's intention and wish to please, the waiter and all others involved, no attempt was made to learn the history, culture, and uniqueness of the customer.

One of the pillars of the theoretical foundation of Psychosomatic People Management is empathy. The concept of empathy is related to the ability to feel what the other person feels, of seeing the situation from the viewpoint of the other, of seeking to relate instantly to the other. Empathy is not the same thing as sympathy. Often we hear people say things like "I really liked so-and-so, I feel great empathy with him." Liking, admiring, wanting to be together or to be friends are related to sympathy, which involves a permanent identification. Examples of permanent identification are the fans of a soccer team, the fans of a singer, those who like and practice a given sport or, also, victims of the same tragedy, who sympathize with each other as they are joined in a cause. The unique characteristic of empathy, on the other hand, is transient identification. It is an ephemeral process, which does not require that people like or have affection or sympathy for someone. It is not necessary to be the same, or even to have experienced what the other did. Empathy is to understand the premises and presuppositions of the other, and only then analyze, process, and act according to the other person's reality. A manager is not born with empathy. The capacity to be empathetic is not taught at school. Once it is understood, it must be practiced. If continuously exercised, it is the most important tool for the modern manager who focuses on aims and results.

Many managers lead their teams in such an aggressive, oppressive, and unintelligent way that they could be called slave drivers, as foremen were called during the time of slavery, who with their tools, the whip and the whipping post, forced slaves to work. Torture was the standard method at the time, and today, surprisingly and unfortunately, torture is still alive and well in many of our companies. Moral harassment has been timidly reported, but it is increasingly the subject of concern of managers, healthcare teams, and lawyers.

In the Wild West films, the American Westerns, we often saw cowboys trying to break the horse that would not stop kicking until they are thrown off. Using spurs and making the horse's hide bleed, the cowboy forcibly inflicted his dominance on the animal. With an iron bit in the mouth, the horse learned that in order not to suffer it had to accept its fate. Many animals, no matter how beautiful and strong nature made them, are rendered useless during the process of forced breaking, and some acquire indelible behavioral flaws that devalue them for trading purposes. Recently, horses began to be tamed using the process of rational breaking, with respect, dedication, and empathy to understand and anticipate the animal's behavior, optimizing the process: greater efficiency and greater productivity at a lower cost.

Psychosomatic People Management is a methodology that uses basic tools. It is very easy to apply and its vital instrument is empathy. In this methodology, the manager and his coworkers should be seen, from the psychological point of view, through a systemic approach, as unique and different beings, even though similar.

A company behaves as a watertight system, often similar to a pressure cooker, and, for the established processes to culminate in the expected result, it must understand that its employees are individuals, with minds that have been formed a long time ago and with strongly rooted behavioral patterns. Psychosomatic People Management proposes that employees should be encouraged to question their role continuously and discuss respect for the dynamism of life, which often is translated into cycles, into different possibilities and aims.

The Axis of Continuous Questioning is the basic tool we have created, and it means to present to employees the relationship of a continuous balance between the static and dynamic aspects of their life roles, be it at work or outside work. Using four apparently simple questions, we encourage them to reflect, always thinking about their development, or to deal with the conflicts that may be present and require rethinking of truths considered absolute and immutable:

1. Who am I?
2. What do I want?
3. Where am I going?
4. How do I get there?

They should be told that there are no single answers to these questions, that it may be good to have multiple answers, that people have multiple roles. But we must help them to choose the best answer for that particular moment in the life history of each person. The discussion should take into account the need to be generous with oneself, to understand that plans made in youth could be the result of immaturity at the time, or, that if there is a conflict between "being what is," and "wanting to be what is not yet," there is time to become it, both from the chronological point of view, and that of Kairós, the inner time, the subjective and relative time that exists in each individual.

Much of the stress that exists in the work environment is caused by the mismatch between desires and aspirations of bosses and the people who report to them. This begins with recruitment and selection processes performed in a rather unintelligent manner, usually by untrained people without the necessary expertise. These processes are often slow and expensive, and do not always pick the right person. This person may even be the most competent, have the best résumé, be the most brilliant, but is not necessarily the most appropriate person for that particular organization. The culture that applicants bring with them may clash directly with the company culture. As in the example of the soccer coach, hired at a very high salary, with a set of enviable benefits, it is possible that even though he is surrounded by a talented team, the new employee withers and does not flourish, and is fired immediately, with a financial burden and wear and tear on all persons involved. After this happens, everyone asks whether, within the company, there was no one who could have been given this managerial position, and whether homegrown talent should really be valued. And the question we ask is: if there were such a person, would he be ready for this?

The greatest hindrance lies precisely in the recruitment and selection processes. A large amount of empathy and much perseverance are needed at this stage, in order to understand and get to know applicants to the utmost, in order to avoid cultural conflicts with the future employer.

Relationships within work teams are another great challenge. Human beings are unique and curiously peculiar creatures. They are greatly bothered by other people's success, but not that of someone unknown or very distant from them. They are bothered by the success of someone who sits next to them, their friend, their neighbor, their relative, and their fellow worker. Human beings are extremely competitive. There is a certain amount of atavism from the time of the caveman, when, in order to survive, it was necessary to dispute the prey with their rivals and always be fully alert, so as not to be devoured by some larger, stronger predator. Strength and speed were key to preserving life. Being efficient was linked to the intuitive capacity to kill in order not to die. In contemporary society there are no more wild beasts devouring us, nor do we have to try our strength against our fellow humans, but envy and competitiveness, now purposeless and possibly sick, undermine the necessary competence to be effective and socially appropriate. Competence is a set of individual attributes essential to performing certain tasks, and they do not presuppose that people should try to be better than others, but rather, that they should do their best.

An extremely competitive individual always has a constant need for self-assertion. This behavior possibly masks a personality with a reasonable level of insecurity, perhaps ill-structured and dysfunctional.

Personality is the result of three constituents, namely: nature, character, and temperament. When an employee does not find it enough to do well, when he needs to know that his co-worker did badly, and only then feels gratified, we have an individual with a dysfunctional personality. This situation is not rare; it must be recognized and identified, and the most appropriate means to deal with this person must be established.

Human beings are full of desires; they desire everything all the time. Ambition and aspirations are legitimate and essential for individual growth and development. However, if the focus of gratification lies not only on doing well, but in doing better than others, or, in an extreme case, wishing that the other does badly, we have here a serious personality problem, often found in the business environment. As an example, let us look at the case of a person who admires Mercedes-Benz cars, and sees several people driving around in the model he desires. Under such circumstances he only feels envy and the wish to have one like it, but if he arrives home and sees the so highly desired car in the neighbor's garage, he feels bad and upset. Possibly he will make jokes at the neighbor's expense, or treat him badly. At a more pathological level, he scratches the neighbor's new car with a key. His sick mind has a psychopathy, since, for him, it is not enough to have the car, which could happen, but the other person who is close to him must not have it. Transferring this issue, to a lesser degree, to a company, we will have fertile ground for envy, hatred, and prejudices in a team that is together for hours and hours, for days and years. All this time together often generates a high dose of familiarity.

If management is mediated by results, they may be achieved, but the question to be asked is, with what quality and at what price? The ingredients that cause stress and a low perception of quality of life at work are there, frolicking around us.

Another crucial aspect to be taken into account is the importance of information and communication in the work environment. Lack of information about internal processes and relevant facts is one of the ingredients of gossip in the halls, and the famous mouth-to-mouth network. The more transparent the communication process is, the better the expected result. Communicating at the right time is another crucial point. Untimely information may be lethal within the business environment. If communication occurs too early, we risk creating a situation of general anxiety, with everyone suffering in advance and becoming incapable of focusing on their work. If communication is late, or if some has already received privileged information, those who should have known it in advance feel left out, devalued, and frustrated.

People tend to look down on the new and unknown. Many changes, including those that meet the needs of coworkers, may be ill received if the manager is not extremely skillful at clearly and objectively communicating what it is all about. A set of information will be received in completely different ways by different employees, and they must have time to think about it and absorb it so that they can internalize and appropriate what is new. In this way, the result of the set is greater that the possible individual difficulties. The focus should always be on communicating at the right time, rapidly and effectively, directly with the person whom the information concerns. In some cases it may be tactically useful to initially go to the coworkers who are opinion-makers. When the communication involves changes that will have a great impact on the group's routine and life, this simple measure ensures better absorption and less rejection of the novelties that are to be implemented.

Psychosomatic People Management assumes that there is a continuous movement of demands and rewards. When the boss demands that the employee do the work for which he was hired, he may say things like "our company is not a charity," "he who pays rules," and so on. If, on the other hand, the boss asked coworkers to cooperate, instead of forcing them to work, that would be a watershed in People Management. What is inherent in cooperation is the request for individuals to fulfill and respect themselves and to give their best, optimizing their time, focusing on the tasks at hand, delivering what they know best and what can be done. By then coworkers will have understood that this is their greatest reward, being respected for their capacity to produce, whether it be a pair of shoes or a quantum physics project. By being respected by their team and by their bosses, and knowing that the result of the entire organization depends on their work, coworkers feel rewarded. At the end of the month, the payment they get is also the confirmation of their skills, competence and feeling of belonging to that group of people.

Appreciation is essential. A thank-you from the boss is very valuable and has the power to heal many traumas, pains, and open wounds that frequently occur in groups of people and are an integral part of life. Managers should show gratitude so their coworkers too can be grateful to the company. This will turn an atmosphere of hostility and friction into one of agreement and peace.

Prizes are a powerful tool to reward good attitudes and good results. If the reward is in money, it will certainly be very useful, but will disappear in the everyday payment of bills, or at the first visit to a shopping mall. More effective rewards occur in the form of providing experiences, moments of delight, something the coworker will never forget. Delighting our fellow man is a process that requires empathy and creativity, possibly that is why it so rarely occurs at our companies. If this delight is also extended to the coworker's family, if there is a concern to make all realize their importance to the company in all processes in which they are involved, the greater will be the coworker's gratification and the company's gain.

Productivity requires motivation. Happiness must be taken into account if the desired targets and results are to be achieved. A conflicted coworker often feels victimized by the company, by his colleagues, and by the management. In that environment, actually nobody is victimizing him, or even wishes him ill. However, for every victim there is a perpetrator, and the workplace, being such an integral part of everyone's life, can very likely become one.

The best coworkers are those who best serve the company's need and have the best relationship with each other. They are the ones who best adapt to the corporate culture; they are more skilled at teamwork; they act proactively and respond rapidly to demands, feeling part of a whole.

Finally, coworkers who present the least conflicts, anxiety, and stress are not those who have the best résumés, the most experienced, those who have been longer with the company, or those who have worked at well-known companies. The coworkers that every manager would like to have in his company are those with a better structured personality, good nature, good character, and good temperament, the kind of person people call the "good guys."

It is not necessary to be friends with ones colleagues, supervisor, or subordinates, but it is essential to be able to trust. An exercise to find out what type of people you have in your team is to ask yourself whether you would be able to entrust your child to them in your absence. But, are there so many people like that around? Is it possible to set up a team which consists only of people like that? The answer to these questions is no. The key here is to know what we should seek in people when we employ them, what values we should encourage in teams, whether it is a janitor or a director. Values are the building blocks of a company, and managing people according to them will make the difference. It is not surprising that today there is so much talk about corporate governance and sustainability, but it cannot only be talk used as corporate advertisement, but rather businesses should walk their talk.

Managers who encourage competitiveness among their subordinates may be generating a hostile and counterproductive atmosphere. We have already discussed the issue of achieving goals at any price and quality.

The level of stress in the work environment begins to be noticed from the high number of medical visits and medical leaves. Somatization conditions become frequent and range from back pain to gastritis and irritable bowel to systemic high blood pressure and coronary syndromes, from headaches to rash. Sleep disorders and libido issues are common complaints. Some of the most commonly diagnosed conditions are anxiety and panic disorders, mood changes, from dysthymia to severe depression, often ending in suicide, as was recently the case at a French company, which called the attention of French health authorities and of all those involved with people management and quality of life at work worldwide.

Changes in the quality of marital relations and family life often go unnoticed in statistics on this subject, but occupational stress may have distant repercussions, leading to imbalance in many members of the worker's family, impacting even their children's performance at school. Reactions can occur in a cascade and in geometrical progression.

Poorly trained or ill-intentioned managers create havoc in the economic situation of the company and of society at large. "Evil" colleagues can undermine the potential of even the best employee if problem detection processes are not permanently on the alert. Furthermore, prevention plans are required to reduce the incidence of these occurrences, because human beings often possess predatory instincts.

The atmosphere of the organization must be systematically evaluated. It is the duty and challenge of modern people managers to keep it as healthy as possible. One must think of smiles as a useful and easily achieved tool for damage prevention, which is one of the aims of Psychosomatic People Management. A focus on damage prevention keeps the company from underestimating the power it has, when poorly guided, to undermine competencies, devalue people, make them ill, or even destroy them.

Joy is a mood that may vary depending on the news you read in the daily papers or what you listen to on the car radio. On the other hand, sadness is part of life. Becoming sad when you lose someone or something you like is part of life and must not be fought with antidepressants. On the other hand, happiness must be understood as a continuous process of human development, where joys and sorrows can be dynamically fitted, where self-esteem is a major factor and depends, among several other factors, on the greater or lesser adaptation and acknowledgment in the work environment.

Psychosomatic People Management is designed to encourage continuous reflection by the company's coworkers, through the Axis of Continuous Questioning that has already been described here. Often it is best for all concerned, once all attempts at training and development of the poorly chosen employee have ceased, to dismiss him, releasing him to find a more appropriate environment according to his history and aspirations.

Everyone at every hierarchical level of the company managed according to the Psychosomatic People Management model should always interact from the viewpoint of the Triadic Action, an intelligent process of action divided into three consecutive phases: perception, working through and acting. During the first phase, perception, the individual must be permanently open, with his perceptive channels clear and unobstructed, to map his surroundings and perceive what happens to others and to himself in relation to the others. The use of all our sensory organs and sensory capacity, which is less and less used by people, should be stimulated.

Next comes the working through stage when the time comes to analyze and understand what was perceived the previous moment and reflect, performing intuitive and rational working through. There is a small unconscious component and a larger conscious one that are used to outline a plan to optimize results, reduce damage, and prevent conflicts. At this stage one should understand and evaluate the situation, keeping in mind the cost/benefit ratio and the pros and cons.

The last phase, called acting, is essential to validate the two previous ones, and focus on movement, on doing, on action proper. It is the time to transform potential, latent energy which exists in plenty in all of us and is stored for long periods, into mechanical energy used to carry out actions. This is when the movement required to preserve the positive state of an individual occurs, or the movement required to make the essential changes needed to maintain well-being.

Triadic Action assumes that to achieve the desired results consistently, it is necessary for the process to occur by experiencing the three phases, independently of how automatic or deeply engrained it already is for some people, while other people must actively embark on it, experience it, and practice it stage by stage.

CHAPTER 13

OCCUPATIONAL STRESS

Causes, Consequences, Prevention and Intervention

Joseph J. Hurrell Jr. and Steven L. Sauter

Occupational stress can be defined as the harmful physical and emotional responses that occur when the requirements of the job do not match the capabilities, resources, or needs of the worker. Stress at work is a prevalent and costly problem in today's workplace. In the U.S., scientific surveys, such as the General Social Survey, have consistently shown high levels of job stress in about one-third of workers during the last two decades (Roper Center for Public Opinion Research, 2007), and a recent survey by the American Psychological Association (American Psychological Association, 2009) found that work was the primary source of stress reported among employed men. Similar findings have been reported in Europe and elsewhere.

Despite recognition by law, medicine, and the insurance industry of the nature of occupational stress, it remains a nebulous construct for many people. While its conceptual roots can be traced to Hans Selye's animal research in the 1930s and Walter Cannon's earlier research on the physiological concomitants of emotion (Quick, Quick, Nelson, & Hurrell, 1997),

Coping and Prevention, pages 231–247

occupational stress as a field of inquiry examining job conditions and their health and performance consequences is a relatively new area of research that crystallized in the early 1970s. The field was given impetus in United States by the establishment of the National Institute for Occupational Safety and Health (NIOSH) and the Occupational Safety and Health Administration (OSHA). The importance of behavioral and motivational factors was acknowledged in provisions of the Occupational Safety and Health Act (OSH Act), which directed NIOSH to include psychological, behavioral, and motivational factors in researching problems of worker safety and health and in developing remedial approaches for these problems. Job-related hazards were interpreted broadly to include conditions of a psychological nature—undue task demands, work conditions, or work regimens that may adversely affect workers' physical or mental health.

NIOSH has sponsored and conducted many research studies that have helped shape the course of job stress research in the United States. For example, in 1988, NIOSH proposed a national strategy for prevention of work-related psychological disorders. Key elements in this prevention strategy include abatement of known job risk factors, research to improve understanding of these risk factors, surveillance to detect and track risk factors, education and training to facilitate recognition of risk factors and their control, and improved mental health services (Sauter, Murphy, & Hurrell, 1990).

In 1996, NIOSH identified "organization of work" as one of the 21 priority research topics for the next decade and developed a comprehensive research agenda for investigating and reducing occupational safety and health risks associated with the rapidly changing nature of work (National Institute for Occupational Safety and Health, 2002). This document described how macro-level forces impact occupational stress. For example, national and international economic, legal, political, technological, and demographic forces influence production methods, human resource policies, management structures, and supervisory practices. These factors, in turn, directly impact the work context, influencing the nature of jobs and the tasks that comprise them. Fueled by global competition, organizational downsizing and restructuring has influenced not only the way work is performed but also—as many laid-off workers can attest—whether work is available to perform.

A MODEL OF JOB STRESS AND HEALTH

Working conditions play a primary role in causing job stress. Exposure to stressful working conditions (job stressors) can have a direct influence on worker safety and health (National Institute for Occupational Safety and

Physical Conditions

Adverse environmental conditions exacerbate overall job demands placed on employees, thus lowering worker tolerance to other stressors and decreasing worker motivation. Environmental conditions, including excessive noise, temperature extremes, poor ventilation, inadequate lighting, and poor ergonomic design have been linked to employee physical and psychological health complaints as well as attitude and behavior problems (see McCoy & Evans, 2005). For example, reports of poor indoor air quality are frequently associated with reports of high levels of job stress. Likewise, outbreaks of psychogenic illness are thought to typically occur in workplaces that employees regard as physically uncomfortable. There is also evidence to suggest that that psychological job stressors produce increments in muscle tension that may exacerbate muscle loads and symptoms resulting from physical demands (Hurrell, 2001).

MODERATING FACTORS

Several personal and situational characteristics can modify the way individual workers exposed to a work environment perceive or react to it. These characteristics, known as "moderators," are depicted in Figure 14.1 in the blocks labeled individual factors, non-work factors, and buffer factors.

Individual Factors

The most widely discussed personal characteristic related to stress at work has been the Type A behavior pattern, characterized by intense striving for achievement, competitiveness, time urgency, excessive drive, and over-commitment to vocation or profession. While investigators in the past have reported the Type A pattern to be independently associated with coronary artery disease, more recent studies have suggested that the variables of hostility, cynicism, anger, irritability, and suspicion may be the primary pathogenic component of the Type A pattern found to be significant in earlier studies. Similarly, while earlier studies suggested an interaction between certain job stressors and Type A characteristics that may lead to heart disease, overall the evidence that Type A persons are more adversely affected by various job stressors is limited.

The hardy personality style and an internal locus of control have been long thought to mediate the stressor–illness relationship. Hardy persons are believed to possess various beliefs and tendencies that are useful in coping with stressors, such as optimistic appraisals of events and decisive actions in coping. Hardy persons report less illness in the presence of stressors. Persons with an internal locus of control—a general belief that events in life are controlled by their actions—also have shown a consistent tendency to report better health than those who believe that life events are beyond their control.

Very recent research from the positive psychology literature has focused on psychological capacity (PsyCap) as a potential mediator of the relationships between exposure to job stressors and health. PsyCap is characterized by confidence, optimism, perseverance, and strong resilience (Luthans, Avolio, Avery, & Norman, 2007). Unlike the earlier notion of the hardy personality, which is generally thought to be trait-like in nature, PsyCap is thought to state-like and therefore more open to change and development.

Factors Outside of Work

Workers do not leave their family and personal problems behind when they go to work, and they do not forget job-related problems on returning home. Nearly all models of job stress acknowledge extra-occupational factors and their potential interaction with work in affecting health outcomes. While some early investigations incorporated generic stressful life events scales into job stress surveys, these scales provided only crude indications of social familial and financial stressors. More recently research interest has focused more specifically on the work family interface. Negative spillover from family to work, positive spillover from family to work, negative spillover from work to family, and positive spillover from work to family have all been documented in the job stress literature. Work and family factors that facilitate development (e.g., job control, family support) have been found to be associated with less negative and more positive spillover between work and family. In contrast, work and family barriers (e.g., job pressure, family disagreements) have been found to be associated with more negative and less positive spillover between work and family (Grzywacz & Marks, 2000).

Work–family conflict has also been of interest to job stress researchers. This is generally conceived of as a situation in which demands from the work and family domains are incompatible in some respect. Such conflict has been found to be associated with work-related consequences (e.g., job satisfaction, organizational commitment, job performance) and non-work-related consequences (e.g., life satisfaction, marital satisfaction) as well as depression and general psychological strain (Allen, Herst, Bruck, & Sutton, 2000).

Buffer Factors

Stress researchers have long sought to identify buffer factors that may reduce or eliminate the effects of job stressors, such as the degree of social support an individual worker receives from work and non-work sources. However, evidence for a buffering effect of social support has been mixed, perhaps due to differences among researchers in conceptualizing and measuring support.

Another potential buffering factor is coping. Coping is a transactional process that is modified continuously by experience within and between stressful episodes. A specific coping strategy that alleviates stress in one situation may not alleviate stress, or may actually increase it, in other situations. Coping responses that people use depend on their social and psychological resources. Social supports and psychological resources, like mastery and self-esteem, are what people draw upon in developing coping strategies. No single coping response is uniformly protective across work and non-work situations. However, having a large and varied coping repertoire can be helpful in reducing stressor–strain relationships. While various coping responses have been found to be effective in the areas of marriage, child rearing, and household finances, coping can be ineffective for work-related problems. This may be due to the impersonal nature of work and the lack of worker control over job stressors.

Lifestyle factors such as physical fitness, and exercise, smoking cessation, and nutrition have the potential to buffer the health effects of job stressors but clear evidence for such buffering is lacking.

PATHOPHYSIOLOGICAL MECHANISMS

Psychological stress is thought to influence a wide range of physiological processes and disease states (Cohen, Janicki-Deverts, & Miller, 2007). However, relatively little is known regarding the specific pathophysiological mechanisms that underlie the relationships between stress and health. Both direct and indirect pathways are thought to play a role. Direct pathways include disregulations of the neurohormonal system (pituitary-adrenocortical axis), the autonomic nervous system, and the immune system. For example, as noted above, rotating shift work influences circadian rhythms, with resultant changes in the autonomic nervous and immune systems. A combination of these pathways, likely influenced by genetic factors, links exposure to job stressors and adverse physical health effects. An indirect pathway links work- and non-work-related stressors to high-risk behaviors and in turn, to adverse health effects. Researchers, for example, have long recognized a strong relationship between stress and substance use and abuse.

Job stressors can also be seen as influencing risk factors for coronary heart disease or triggers for acute myocardial infarction. Acutely, stress increases catecholamine levels, leading to increased heart rate and blood pressure, decreased plasma volume, coronary constriction, and increased lipid levels, platelet activity, coagulation, and inflammation. Chronically, stress causes autonomic imbalance, neurohormonal changes (such as elevated cortisol and norepinephrine levels), a pro-coagulant state (characterized by blood hypercoaguabiligy), and increased lipid levels. Immune system responses may mediate some of these relationships. Animal studies have demonstrated that experimentally induced stress increases susceptibility to various infectious agents and the incidence and rate of growth of lymphomas and ovarian pulmonary tumors. Some human studies have shown that psychosocial factors, including stressful life events, are related to immunological disorders such as asthma, allergies, and autoimmune diseases. And stress has been linked to changes in levels of circulating antibodies, lymphocytic cytotoxicity, and lymphocyte proliferation.

PREVENTION AND INTERVENTION

The gap between etiologic and intervention-related knowledge in the realm of occupational stress is great. Despite the ever-burgeoning literature on the nature, causes, and physical and psychological consequences of occupational stress, surprisingly little is known about intervention for occupational stress. Views differ regarding the importance of worker characteristics versus working conditions as "the" major cause of organizational stress; these views have, in part, led to the development and use of primary, secondary, and tertiary prevention (intervention) approaches for occupational stress. The aim of primary prevention intervention is to reduce risk factors or job stressors. The aim of secondary prevention intervention for occupational stress is to alter the ways that individuals respond to risks or job stressors. And the aim of tertiary prevention intervention is to heal those who have been traumatized. These three aims are depicted in Figure 14.1. Research on primary and tertiary prevention intervention has been reviewed by Hurrell (2005) and Kelloway, Hurrell, and Day (2008), while secondary prevention intervention has been the subject of reviews by Murphy (1996) and van der Klink and colleagues (van der Klinck, Blonk, Schene, & van Dijk, 2001). The following provides a brief overview of research findings for all three types of intervention.

Primary Prevention Interventions

Although generally thought to be the most effective approach to dealing with work stress, primary prevention interventions are one of the least studied areas of work stress. Primary prevention interventions can be characterized as either psychosocial or socio-technical. Psychosocial interventions focus primarily on human processes and psychosocial aspects of the work setting and aim to reduce stress by changing workers' perceptions of the work environment; they may also include modifications of objective working conditions. In contrast, socio-technical interventions focus primarily on changes to objective working conditions and are considered to have implications for work-related stress. Some interventions involve elements of both approaches.

Most primary prevention interventions appear to be psychosocial. Many are based upon the principles of participatory action research (PAR), in which researchers and workers collaborate in a process of data-guided problem solving to improve the organization's ability to provide workers with desired outcomes and to contribute to general operational knowledge. Participatory action research involves workers and experts from outside the workplace in an empowering process of defining problems (identifying stressors), developing intervention strategies, introducing changes that benefit employees, and measuring outcomes. Some PAR interventions have specifically focused on efforts to redesign work or work processes. In general, there is very limited evidence for the efficacy of PAR and other participatory-type interventions; studies evaluating its efficacy tend to be methodologically weak, difficult to interpret, and causally ambiguous. When found, the effects of the interventions have often been on job satisfaction and perceptions of the working environment; few effects on health-related outcomes have been reported. It is unclear whether the general lack of health benefits are due to ineffective interventions, the insufficient duration of the studies, or the nature of the health-outcome variables studied. Moreover, which effects are attributable to the act of participating in the intervention and which are attributable to changes in working conditions or processes resulting from the intervention are unclear.

There is, however, some evidence for the efficacy of psychosocial interventions focused upon supervisors and managers, rather than workers. While few in number, these interventions resulted in positive organizationally relevant outcomes and found modest positive effects on individual well-being. An intriguing aspect is that the effects on well-being may extend beyond the supervisors and managers themselves, possibly representing a potentially effective and seemingly cost-efficient approach to primary prevention. No firm conclusions, however, can be drawn.

In contrast to psychosocial interventions, socio-technical interventions are generally not a result of employee–employer or employee–employer–researcher collaboration. Socio-technical interventions have generally involved changing only a very limited variety of objective working conditions, such as workloads, work schedules, and work processes. However, as a whole, socio-technical intervention studies provide more consistent and robust evidence for the efficacy of the intervention than psychosocial intervention studies. In addition to incorporating self-report measures of affect, such as job satisfaction, anxiety, and depression, most of these studies have incorporated objective outcome measures, such as blood pressure, job performance, and sickness absence, in the study design. In general, these studies have also tended to utilize more rigorous experimental and quasi-experimental designs.

Secondary Prevention Interventions

Secondary interventions generally focus on altering the relationship between stressors and strains by either increasing individual resilience to stress (e.g., through health promotion) or by teaching specific techniques to address the symptoms of strain (e.g., stress-management training). Perhaps ironically, secondary interventions are often thought to be less effective, but implemented more frequently in organizations, than are primary interventions. Secondary interventions may be less effective because they are either too general (i.e., not targeted toward a particular experience) and are invoked only after the stress has occurred. Moreover, these types of individual-level interventions do not tend to have long-term organizational or individual health benefits, perhaps because they don't facilitate long-term behavioral changes. Despite these criticisms, secondary interventions are often chosen over primary prevention interventions because the costs and logistics are thought to be less excessive.

Wellness initiatives offered in the workplace (generally under the rubric of health promotion) typically focus on lifestyle factors such as smoking, nutrition, exercise, and blood pressure control. Although there is mixed evidence for the success of such interventions, there is little doubt that they are popular among employees and appear to be gaining acceptance in industry. Evidence regarding the efficacy of such interventions could result from a current NIOSH initiative (NIOSH WorkLife) launched in 2004, which is facilitating collaboration between health and safety professionals and health promotion specialists to develop and implement workplace programs that prevent occupational illness and injury, promote health, and optimize the health of workers. A major premise of this initiative is that comprehensive practices and policies that consider both the physical work environment and the organizational work environment, while addressing personal health risks of workers, are more effective in preventing disease and promoting health and safety than each approach is separately.

Stress management training (SMT) involves a wide variety of techniques and procedures designed to help workers modify their appraisal of stressful situations and/or to deal with the symptoms of stress. Typically, such interventions are prescriptive, person-oriented, relaxation-based techniques, such as biofeedback, progressive muscle relaxation, meditation, and cognitive–behavioral skills training. They differ from other health-promotion programs in the variety of training techniques and wide range of health-outcome measures used to assess program effectiveness. In contrast to primary prevention interventions, they do not seek to alter the sources of stress at work (job stressors) through organizational change strategies or job redesign. There is evidence for the effectiveness of such programs, although some of these effects may be only short-term. In contrast to research on health promotion activities, in which the evidence may be more equivocal, the data generally support the implementation of stress-management programs for the reduction of worker stress.

Cognitive–behavioral skills training, frequently used in stress management, involves techniques designed to modify the appraisal processes that determine perceived stressfulness of situations and to develop behavioral skills for managing stressors. It helps people to restructure their thinking patterns through cognitive restructuring. In general, it can reduce psychological strain, especially anxiety, and improve organizationally relevant outcomes such as job satisfaction. However, it has not shown consistent improvement of physiological strains.

In contrast, muscle relaxation techniques can benefit some physiological strains, such as blood pressure, but not others. Such techniques involve focusing one's attention on muscle activity, learning to identify even small amounts of tension in a muscle group, and practicing releasing of tension from muscles.

Meditation methods used in worksite stress-management studies, often secular versions of transcendental meditation, involve sitting upright in a comfortable position, in a quiet place, with eyes closed, and mentally repeating a mantra while maintaining a passive attitude. The few studies that have examined the efficacy of such worksite-based meditation provide consistent evidence that they reduce psychological, physiological, and behavioral strain.

Combinations of two or more stress-management approaches into a single intervention are quite common. The most common combination and most effective seems to be muscle relaxation coupled with cognitive–behavioral skills training.

Tertiary Prevention Interventions

In contrast to the secondary focus on treating the short-term symptoms of stress, tertiary interventions are focused on treating the physical, psychological, or behavioral consequences of exposures to job stressors. The following is a brief overview of these interventions.

Many large companies have occupational medicine departments that offer services that include urgent medical care, employee examinations, disability reviews, health promotion activities, and referrals for medical treatment. In general, these departments are not structured to provide extensive or long-term care for stress-related illness or injury and must rely on making referrals to appropriate health-care providers. Mental health problems related to job stress can present special challenges to occupational medicine departments that may not be well equipped either to deal with them or to make referrals.

Counseling and psychotherapy are commonly used methods to treat individuals suffering from work-related mental health problems. Common techniques of psychotherapy and counseling include behavioral and cognitive therapy, supportive counseling, and insight-oriented psychotherapy. Counseling and psychotherapy can have marked benefits on symptom reduction, but they may not have a beneficial impact on work performance (as measured by reduced absenteeism).

Many companies offer limited counseling at the workplace through employee assistance programs (EAPs) that often provide a variety of mental health-related services. Employees can refer themselves to EAPs or be referred by management. The goals of EAPs are to restore employees to full productivity by (1) identifying those with drug abuse, and those with emotional or behavioral problems that result in deficient work performance; (2) motivating these employees to seek help; (3) providing short-term professional counseling assistance and referral; (4) directing employees toward the best assistance available; and (5) providing continuing support and guidance throughout the problem-solving period. Very few studies have addressed the cost-effectiveness of individual EAPs. There is little agreement on evaluation methodology. And some have questioned whether there should be any economic evaluation of EAPs. However, reduced health claims, financial savings, lower absenteeism rates, and increased return on investment have been reported.

For many employees, a stigma continues to be associated with psychological treatment of any kind. This fear, along with concerns regarding confidentiality, may limit the use of workplace-based mental health resources. Employees may also feel that the company has a vested interest in their productivity that is of greater importance than their health. This concern may be exacerbated by EAPs being gatekeepers with financial incentives to not refer employees for more sophisticated and long-term care and instead refer them to mental health care providers with limited training who may charge the employer less money. Psychologists, psychiatrists, and social workers seem to achieve equally positive outcomes, whereas other counseling professionals who generally charge less money do not appear to achieve outcomes as positive. There are paradoxes embedded in the very nature of

EAPs, which lead to conflicting demands and occupational stress for EAP professionals, such as pressures to provide short-term individual solutions to what may be long-term structural problems (Bento, 1997).

Implications for Practice

A tremendous gulf exists between our knowledge regarding job stress and the most efficacious and economical means of preventing it and treating its consequences in the workplace. There is only limited evidence that certain primary prevention interventions have worked. Those that focus on a few stressors and those that do not introduce too many changes too quickly appear to be the most successful. Before primary prevention interventions are designed and implemented, the most prevalent and problematic stressors must be identified and prioritized according to their potency and amenability to meaningful change (Hurrell & Murphy, 1996). Practitioners and researchers should target appropriate objective and subjective outcomes for assessing the efficacy of interventions as well as valid and reliable measures of these outcomes. Objective measures that are organizationally relevant need to be included, without which other organizations will be reluctant to implement these interventions.

Job stress interventions are all too often implemented in relative isolation from one another within an organization. For example, management, human resources, the medical departments, and/or the EAP may be given the responsibility for an intervention, and there may be little involvement or cooperation with other organizational structures. Any and all interventions for job stress should be integrated within the organization as a whole.

Given that each intervention may not be possible or effective for all stressors, a comprehensive approach to the issue of job stress should include all three forms of intervention. Pragmatically, the only way that organizations can reduce risks of occupational stress and resulting organizational costs is to implement effective programs aimed at primary intervention, buffering or remediation (secondary intervention), and treatment (tertiary prevention).

REFERENCES

Allen, T. D., Herst, D. E. L., Bruck, C. S., & Sutton, M. (2000). Consequences associated with work to family conflict: A review and agenda for the future. *Journal of Occupational Health Psychology, 5*, 278–308.

American Psychological Association. (2009). *Stress in America 2009.* Washington, DC: American Psychological Association.

Bakker, A. B., & Demerouti, E. (2007). The job demands–resources model: State of the art. *Journal of Managerial Psychology, 22*, 309–328.

Barling, J., Kelloway, E. K., & Frone, M. R. (Eds.). (2004). *Handbook of work stress.* Thousand Oaks, CA: Sage.

Belkic, K. Landsbergis, P., Schnall, P., & Baker, D. (2004). Is job strain a major source of cardiovascular disease risk? *Scandinavian Journal of Work Environment and Health,* 30, 85–128.

Bento, R. F. (1997). On the other hand . . . the paradoxical nature of employee assistance programs. *Employee Assistance Quarterly, 13,* 83–91.

Cohen, S., Janicki-Deverts, D., & Miller, G. E. (2007). Psychological stress and disease. *Journal of the American Medical Association, 298,* 1685–1687.

Goetzel R. Z., Anderson, D. R., Whitmer, R. W., Ozminkowski, R. J., Dunn, R. L., & Wasserman, J. (1998). The relationship between modifiable health risks and health care expenditures: An analysis of the multi-employer HERO health risk and cost database. *Journal of Occupational and Environmental Medicine, 40,* 843–854.

Grzywacz , J., & Marks, N. F. (2000). Reconceptualizing the work–family interface: An ecological perspective on the correlates of positive and negative spillover between work and family. *Journal of Occupational Health Psychology, 5,* 111–126.

Hurrell, J. J. Jr. (2001). Psychosocial factors and musculoskeletal disoreders. In P. Perrewé & D. Ganster (Eds.), *Exploring theoretical mechanisms and perspectives: Research in occupational stress and well-being* (Vol. 1, pp. 233–256). New York, NY: Elsevier.

Hurrell, J. J., Jr. (2005). Occupational stress intervention. In E. Kelloway, J. Barling, & M. Frone (Eds.), *Handbook of stress* (pp. 623–645). Thousand Oaks, CA: Sage.

Hurrell, J. J., Jr. & Murphy, L.R. (1996). Occupational stress intervention. *American Journal of Industrial Medicine, 29,* 338–341.

Karasek, R. A., & Theorell T. (1990). *Healthy work: Stress, productivity, and the reconstruction of working life.* New York, NY: Basic Books.

Kelloway, E. K. Barling, J., & Hurrell J. J., Jr. (Eds.). (2006). *Workplace violence.* Thousand Oaks, CA: Sage.

Kelloway, E. K., Hurrell, J. J., Jr., & Day, A. (2008). Workplace interventions for occupational stress. In K. Naswall, M. Sverke, & J. Hellgren (Eds.), *The Individual in the changing workplace* (pp. 419–442). Cambridge, UK: Cambridge University Press.

Lerner, D., Adler, D. A., Chang, H., Berndt, E. R., Irish, J. T., Lapitsky, L . . . Rogers, W.H. (2004). The clinical and occupational correlates of work productivity loss among employed patients with depression. *Journal of Occupational and Environmental Medicine, 46,* S46–S55.

Lerner, D., Adler, D. A., Rogers, W. H. Hong, C., Lapitsky, L., McLaughlin, T. & Reed, J. (2010). Work performance of employees with depression: The impact of work stressors. *American Journal of Health Promotion, 24,* 205–213.

Luthans, F., Avolio, B. J., Avery, J. B. & Norman, S. M. (2007). Positive psychological capital: Measurement and relationship with performance and satisfaction. *Personnel Psychology, 60,* 541–572.

McCoy, J. M., & Evans, G. (2005). Physical work environment. In J. Barling, E. K. Kelloway, & M. Frone (Eds.), *Handbook of work* (pp. 219–245). Thousand Oaks, CA: Sage.

Murphy, L. R. (1996). Stress management in work settings: a critical review of the health effects. *American Journal of Health Promotion, 11,* 112–135.

National Institute for Occupational Safety and Health. (1997). *Plain language about shiftwork.* [DHHS (NIOSH) Publication No. 97-145]. Washington, DC: US Government Printing Office.

National Institute for Occupational Safety and Health. (1999). *Stress at work.* [DHHS (NIOSH) Publication No. 99-101]. Washington, DC: U.S. Government Printing Office.

National Institute for Occupational Safety and Health. (2002). *The changing organization of work and safety and the health of working people: knowledge gaps and research directions.* [DHHS (NIOSH) Publication No. 2002-116]. Washington, DC: U.S. Government Printing Office.

National Institute for Occupational Safety and Health. (2004). *Overtime and extended work shifts: recent findings on illness, injuries and health behaviors.* [DHHS (NIOSH) Publication No. 2004-143]. Washington, DC: U.S. Government Printing Office.

Netterstrom, B., Conrad, N., Bech, P., Fink, P., Olsen, O., Rugulies, R., & Stansfeld, S. (2008). The relation between work-related psychosocial factors and the development of depression. *Epidemiologic Reviews, 30,* 118–132.

Quick, J. C., Quick, J. D., Nelson, D. L., & Hurrell, J. J., Jr. (1997). *Preventive stress management in organizations.* Washington, DC: American Psychological Association.

Roper Center for Public Opinion Research. (2007, March). *General social surveys, 1972–2006: Cumulative codebook.* Storrs, CT: Author.

Sauter, S. L., Hurrell. J. J., Jr, & Cooper, C. L. (Eds.). (1989). *Job control and worker health.* Chichester, UK: John Wiley & Sons.

Sauter, S. L.,, Murphy, L. R., & Hurrell, J. J., Jr. (1990). Prevention of work-related psychological disorders: a national strategy proposed by the National Institute for Occupational Safety and Health (NIOSH). *American Psychologist, 45,* 1146–1158.

Siegrist J. (1996). Adverse health effects of high/low reward conditions. *Journal of Occupational Health Psychology, 8,* 27–41.

Van der Klinck J. J. L., Blonk, R. W. B., Schene, A. H., & van Dijk, F. J. (2001). The benefits of interventions for work-related stress. *American Journal of Public Health, 91,* 270–276.

Van Vaqchel, N., de Jonge, J., Bosma, H., & Schaufeli, W. (2005). Reviewing the effort–reward imbalance model: Drawing up the balance of 45 empirical studies. *Social Science and Medicine, 60,* 1117–1131.

ABOUT THE CONTRIBUTING AUTHORS

Interpersonal Conflict and Stress at Work: Implications for Employee Health and Well-Being

Valentina Bruk-Lee is assistant professor of industrial/organizational psychology at Florida International University. Her research is primarily focused on the topics of interpersonal conflict in organizations, occupational well-being, job stress, and new mothers returning to employment. Her work has been published in peer-reviewed journals and presented at national conferences. She has consulted with both private and public-sector organizations in the areas of employee selection, job analysis, performance measurement, and competency modeling.

Paul E. Spector is a distinguished university professor of industrial/organizational (I/O) psychology and I/O doctoral program director at the University of South Florida. He is also director of the NIOSH-funded Sunshine Education and Research Center's Occupational Health Psychology program. He is the Associate Editor for Point/Counterpoint for *Journal of Organizational Behavior* and Associate Editor for *Work & Stress*; he is is on the editorial boards of *Journal of Applied Psychology*, *Organizational Research Methods*, and *Personnel Psychology*.

Coping and Prevention, pages 249–255

Organizational Identity, Social Support Systems, and Occupational Stress: The Development of a Conceptual Model

Jason Stoner joined the College of Business at Ohio University in 2007. Dr. Stoner completed his PhD in Organizational Behavior and Human Resource Management at Florida State University. His research interests are in the areas of organizational stress and identity, primarily focusing on individual differences influencing individuals' reactions to workplace stressors. Dr. Jason Stoner's research has been published in *Human Relations, Human Resource Management Review, Leadership Quarterly, Journal of Occupational and Health Psychology,* and *Journal of Vocational Behavior.*

Pamela L. Perrewé (PhD) is the Haywood and Betty Taylor Eminent Scholar of Business Administration and Distinguished Research Professor at Florida State University. Dr. Perrewé has published several books, over 20 book chapters, and over 100 journal articles in journals such as *Academy of Management Journal, Journal of Management, Journal of Applied Psychology,* and *Organizational Behavior and Human Decision Processes.*

The Relationship Between Alcohol Use and Work

Edilaine C. Silva Gherardi-Donato is a professor at the Nursing School of Ribeirão Preto, Department of Psychiatric Nursing and Human Sciences at the University of São Paulo, PhD in Nursing, researcher in the use of psychoactive substances and stress.

Margarita Antonia Villar Luis is a professor at the Nursing School of Ribeirão Preto, Department of Psychiatric Nursing and Human Sciences at the University of São Paulo, PhD in Nursing, researcher in the use of psychoactive substances and stress.

Clarissa Mendonça Corradi-Webster is a Psychologist, PhD in Psychology, researcher at the University of São Paulo.

Age-Related Trends in Workers' Subjective Well-Being and Perceived Job Quality

Jessica M. Streit is a Research Psychologist in the National Institute for Occupational Safety and Health (NIOSH)'s Division of Applied Research and Technology. Her current research projects are quite diverse and address topics such as alternative break schedules, office ergonomics, best practices for scientific information dissemination, and methods to culturally adapt and validate research tools. Jessica also teaches undergraduate-level industrial/organizational psychology courses for Northern Kentucky University's Department of Psychological Sciences. Presently, she is pursuing graduate-level studies in the fields of predictive analytics and data mining.

Steven Sauter is a consultant to the National Institute for Occupational Safety and Health where he formerly served as Coordinator of the NIOSH Program on Work Organization and Stress. He presently serves as one of the Associate Editors of the Journal of Occupational Health Psychology.

Dennis Hanseman is a biostatistician and consultant in the Department of Surgery, University of Cincinnati College of Medicine. He undertakes observational studies and clinical trials in the areas of surgery, neuropsychiatry, and health services research. He is a member of the American Statistical Association and the Society for Epidemiologic Research.

Social Reward and Health—How to Reduce Stress at Work and Beyond

Johannes Siegrist is Professor and Director of the Department of Medical Sociology and Director of the Public Health Program at the University of Duesseldorf. His main research areas are: adverse health effects of psychosocial stress at work (development of the Effort-Reward-Imbalance model) and social determinants of health in early old age. He is Associate Editor or member of the Advisory Board of several international journals including *International Journal of Behavioral Medicine* and *Work & Stress.*

That Wasn't Too Stressful, or Was It: Physiological Stress Responses to Regulatory Focus (Mis)Match

Chad Ian Peddie is a Research Associate in the Personnel Selection and Development Program of the Human Resources Research Organization. He graduated with both a bachelor's degree in psychology and a master's degree in industrial/organizational psychology from George Mason University. He has conducted research in organizational demography, diversity training, workplace discrimination, employee selection, and occupational health psychology. His work has been published in peer-reviewed journals, book chapters, and presented at national conferences.

Julie A. Agar is an Associate Human Capital Consultant at PDRI. In addition to human capital consulting, she also has considerable experience in health care research and is interested in the intersection between these two fields. Ms. Agar completed her Master's degree in Industrial/Organizational Psychology from George Mason University.

Kate A. LaPort is a Research Psychologist in the Personnel Assessment Research Unit at the U.S. Army Research Institute for the Behavioral and Social Sciences. She is a doctoral candidate in the I/O Psychology program at George Mason University. Her research interests include noncognitive assessments, examining patterns of leader traits, and leader emotion management.

Lois E. Tetrick is the Director of the Industrial and Organizational Psychology Program at George Mason University. She co-edited the *Handbook of Occupational Health Psychology* (1st and 2nd editions) with James Campbell Quick. Dr. Tetrick's interests are in stress, work and family issues, occupational safety, and positive emotions in the workplace, especially as they affect employee and organizational health.

The Relationship between Family-Supportive Culture, Work-Family Conflict, and Emotional Exhaustion: A Multilevel Study

Kristi Zimmerman is a Research Associate at Pacific Research and Evaluation and received her Ph.D. from Portland State University in 2009. Her research interests focus on the relationship between work–family conflict health and safety outcomes. Her work focuses on evaluating training and professional development programs in school districts and non-profit organizations.

Leslie B. Hammer is a Professor of Psychology in the Department of Psychology at Portland State University. Her research focuses on ways in which organizations can help reduce work and family stress and improve positive spillover by facilitating both formal and informal workplace supports. She is the Director of the Center for Work–Family Stress, Safety, and Health, funded by a federal grant.

Tori Crain is a PhD candidate in the Applied Psychology Program at Portland State University. She is pursuing a degree in Industrial/Organizational Psychology with an emphasis in Occupational Health Psychology. Her research interests focus on the relationship between employees' work–family conflict and objective health outcomes. She is a research assistant at the Center for Work–Family Stress, Safety, and Health.

Stress Management and Occupational Quality of Life Programs in Public Security

Tatiana Severino de Vasconcelos earned a PhD in Social and Occupational Psychology from the University of Brasília, expert in Public Policies and Government Management with the Federal Administration, currently in charge of the Project Quality of Life for public security professionals at SENASP—Brazilian Ministry of Justice.

Quality of Life and Burnout in Physicians

Avelino Luiz Rodrigues is a professor in the Department of Clinical Psychology at the University of São Paulo (IPUSP); coordinator of the Subject and Body Laboratory with IPUSP (SUCOR); honorary member of the Brazilian Association of Psychosomatic Medicine; leader of the CNPq research group: Psychosomatics, Psychoneurology and Health Promotion; Physician.

Elisa Maria Parahyba Campos is associate professor in the Department of Clinical Psychology of the Institute of Psychology, São Paulo University (IPUSP); founder of the Brazilian Society of Psycho-Oncology; coordinator of the Laboratory and Humanistic Center for Cancer Recovery and Health (CHRONOS), member of the CNPq research group: Psychosomatics, Psychoneurology and Health Promotion; clinical psychologist.

Guilherme Borges Valente is a master student in Clinical Psychology at IPUSP, member of the Subject and Body Laboratory with IPUSP (SUCOR); member of the CNPq research group: Psychosomatics, Psychoneurology and Health Promotion; clinical psychologist.

Healthy Possibilities to Face a Hypermodern Life: Different Facets of Constructive Spare Time

Ieda Rhoden has a PhD in Spare Time and Human Potential (University of Deusto/Spain); master in Business Administration (PUC-RI); psychologist (PUCRS). Professor at UNISINOS for 20 years and consultant in People Management and Quality of Life. For ten years she has been studying the subjective experiences of enjoyment and self-development in spare time and at work.

"Not so Fast, my Friend": The Eternal Marital Bliss or Imminent Divorce of Leadership and Neuroscience

Thomas A. Zeni is a doctoral student in Industrial & Organizational Psychology at the University of Oklahoma. He holds a Master of Science degree in I/O Psychology from the University of Oklahoma, and is a certified Professional in Human Resources (PHR). His research interests include emotions in organizations, individual differences, counterproductive work behaviors, and psychometric methods.

M. Ronald Buckley (PhD, Auburn University) is the JC Penney Company Chair of Business Leadership and a Professor of Management and Professor of Psychology in the Price College of Business at the University of Oklahoma. His primary research interests are in traditional Human Resources Management topics, but he has, on occasion, published articles in other organizational sciences topics.

Anthony C. Klotz is a doctoral student in organizational behavior in the Price College of Business at the University of Oklahoma. He has a Master of Business Administration degree from Creighton University. His research interests include organizational citizenship behavior, counterproductive work behavior, impression management, and team conflict.

Milorad M. Novicevic (PhD, University of Oklahoma) is an Associate Professor of Management at the University of Mississippi. His research focuses on management history and international management. He has published more than 100 articles in various journals including the *Leadership Quarterly, Human Resource Management,* and *Organization Behavior and Human Decision Processes.*

People Management: A Psychosomatic View

Artur Zular is a scientific consultant with the Instituto Qualidade de Vida, president of the Psychosomatic Medicine Committee with the São Paulo Medical Association, vice-president of ABMP-SP and former chief professor of the Psychosomatic Medicine course at the Santo Amaro Medical School. Professor of specialization programs on Psychology and Occupational Quality of Life at PUCSP and IQV.

Occupational Stress: Causes, Consequences, Prevention, and Intervention

Joseph J. Hurrell Jr., is the current editor of the *Journal of Occupational Health Psychology* (*JOHP*) and was previously affiliated with the U.S. National Institute for Occupational Safety and Health (NIOSH), where he authored over 120 publications on job stress. Dr. Hurrell was also a founding member of the Society for Occupational Health Psychology.

Steven Sauter is a consultant to the National Institute for Occupational Safety and Health where he formerly served as Coordinator of the NIOSH Program on Work Organization and Stress. He presently serves as one of the Associate Editors of the Journal of Occupational Health Psychology.

Printed and bound by CPI Group (UK) Ltd, Croydon, CR0 4YY

15/09/2026

14962368-0005